Renal Pathophysiology

Avery R. Harrington, M.D.

Associate Professor of Medicine
University of Wisconsin–Madison

Stephen W. Zimmerman, M.D.

Associate Professor of Medicine and Pathology
University of Wisconsin–Madison

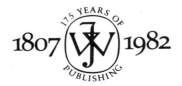

175 YEARS OF PUBLISHING

1807 1982

A WILEY MEDICAL PUBLICATION

JOHN WILEY & SONS / **New York • Chichester • Brisbane • Toronto**

B + T   9-13-83

Cover design by Wanda Lubelska
Production Editor: Cheryl Howell

The cover photo of a scanning electron micrograph is reproduced with permission from P. M. Burkholder, **Atlas of Human Glomerular Pathology,** *New York, Harper & Row, 1974.*

Library of Congress Cataloging in Publication Data:
Harrington, Avery R.
  Renal pathophysiology.
  Includes bibliographical references and index.
  1. Kidneys. 2. Kidneys—Diseases. 3. Physiology.
Pathological. I. Zimmerman, Stephen W. II. Title.
[DNLM: 1. Kidney—Physiopathology. WJ 300 H299r]
QP249.H36   616.6'1   81-7454
ISBN 0-471-07815-8   AACR2

Printed in the United States of America

10 9 8 7 6 5 4 3 2 1

To Carolyn and Jan, who gave up a great deal of love and companionship so that we could write this book

Series Preface

It has come to be generally appreciated that knowledge concerning the pathophysiology of organ dysfunction serves as the basis for our understanding of the underlying mechanisms of disease. The phenomenal growth of pathophysiology as a discipline during the past ten years and its efficacy in medical education have prompted the preparation of the Wiley Pathophysiology Series.

Until recently, the traditional method of instructing first- and second-year medical students has been to teach the basic sciences including pharmacology and biochemistry separately. Today, however, an increasing number of medical schools have come to favor a multidisciplinary course of study where the pathophysiology of each organ system is examined and dealt with in its entirety. It has been found that this provides medical students with a firm base of knowledge concerning cellular biology and basic science and their relevance to the practice of medicine. The purpose of this series is to offer an accompaniment to such a curriculum that is both thorough and up-to-date.

The first book in the series, *Pathophysiology of Respiration* deals with the disordered function of the respiratory system. Dr. Kryger and his colleagues at the University of Manitoba Medical School present a concise multidisciplinary treatment of the subject that touches on all aspects of the altered performance of the diseased lung. It is felt that this work adds a valuable perspective to current medical knowledge, and it is hoped that teachers and practitioners of medicine as well as second-year students will find it stimulating and useful.

The unfailing support and courtesy of the staff of John Wiley & Sons is gratefully acknowledged.

Neville Bittar, M.D.
University of Wisconsin, Madison

Preface

In our contacts with second-year medical students we have often been impressed by their ability to learn large amounts of detailed material in a short time—a talent that serves them well in the early years of their medical education. When we deal with more advanced students and medical residents, however, we are sometimes chagrined to discover that some fundamental principles of renal physiology and disease have escaped them. All of us have difficulty remembering many of the things we have learned. But perhaps a part of the problem here is that the original learning was focused too much on numerous facts to be remembered and not enough on basic concepts.

This book attempts to address that problem by emphasizing the basic ideas in current knowledge of renal physiology and disease. We have presented these ideas in an informal style that we hope is lucid, interesting, and even entertaining at times. Of course, there is far more to be learned about renal physiology and disease than what we have included. It is our hope that at least some readers will become sufficiently interested in the subject to pursue it elsewhere in more detail. We have not attempted to provide references to original experimental work, but we have listed at the end of each chapter some general review articles or other sources where the student may find more information and references.

A more detailed and scholarly approach than ours may also be found in a number of other texts. Among these, we should mention especially the classic by Robert F. Pitts, *Physiology of the Kidney and Body Fluids* (Chicago: Year Book Medical Publishers, 3rd ed., 1974), and two books by Heinz Valtin, *Renal Function* (Boston: Little, Brown, 1973) and *Renal Dysfunction* (Boston: Little, Brown, 1979). Our readers should also be aware of the big books—multiauthored volumes whose editors have succeeded in pulling together much of what is currently known about kidneys. The most available and recently published of these are *Strauss and Welt's Diseases of the Kidney*, edited by L. E. Earley and C. W. Gottschalk (Third Edition, Little, Brown & Co., 1979); *The Kidney*, edited by B. M. Brenner and F. C. Rector, Jr. (Second Edition, W. B. Saunders Co., 1981); *Nephrology*, edited by J. Hamburger, J. Crosnier, and J. P. Grünfeld (John Wiley & Sons, 1979); and *Pediatric Kidney Disease*, edited by C. M. Edelmann, Jr. (Little, Brown & Co., 1978). These volumes provide abundant detail about almost everything renal and are therefore fine reference sources, but they may be difficult reading for a newcomer to the field.

Although this book deals primarily with pathology and normal and abnormal physiology, we have included some clinical material where it seemed appropriate, especially in the last six chapters. We have devoted two of those chapters to basic discussions of dialysis and renal transplantation because the management of patients with renal failure in the developed world now depends heavily on these methods; moreover, students often find themselves dealing with such patients without any introduction to the principles underlying their treatment.

We are enthusiastically in favor of sexual equality, but the English language does not provide a singular pronoun that refers to a person of either gender. "He or she" is too clumsy for repeated use, so we have reluctantly adopted the convention of using "he" for a person whose sex is not specified. We hope that our readers will interpret this as "he or she."

We would like to express our indebtedness to the many persons whose help and encouragement made this book possible. Many of our professional colleagues at the University of Wisconsin–Madison provided information, made suggestions, or reviewed chapters for us; they include Judith Blank, A. Vishnu Moorthy, Terry Oberley, David Simpson, Thomas Steele, Stuart Updike, Arvin Weinstein, and Sung-Feng Wen. Peter Burkholder did the electron microscopy on the renal biopsy specimens that are illustrated in the book. Michael Madden, a fellow in Nephrology, did most of the research and much of the writing in the chapters on dialysis and renal transplantation. He also reviewed several other chapters. A number of our second-year medical students (who were guinea pigs for some of these chapters) made useful suggestions and encouraged us to continue with this project.

Sue Reckinger and Avis Steele provided general secretarial support, and Linda Croxford, Lori Stalsberg, and especially Donna Davis did extensive typing, retyping, and correcting of the manuscript. Barbara Goodsit was responsible for almost all the original drawings. The diligence and patience of these women was greatly appreciated.

The preparation of this book placed unusual burdens on our wives, whose understanding support enabled us to continue. In addition, Carolyn Harrington spent many hours perusing the manuscript in order to help us eliminate nebulous writing. She also contributed one of the drawings.

Avery R. Harrington
Stephen W. Zimmerman

Contents

Renal
Pathophysiology

1
Some Basic Ideas

Not everyone who reads this book will start with the same background of information. So where should we begin? We would like this text to be understandable to everyone with a basic knowledge of physiology and biological chemistry, but we do not want to bore our readers with a recitation of what many of them already know. As a compromise we shall devote this chapter to a brief discussion of several concepts which are important to an understanding of subjects to be presented later. Those who are already well acquainted with this introductory material may choose to skip over it.

BODY FLUID COMPARTMENTS

Water accounts for 50 to 70% of the human body by weight. The variation is explained largely by individual differences in body fat content. Adipose tissue may contribute heavily to body weight, but it contains only about 10% water. Muscle tissue, on the other hand, contains about 75% water. The finding that total body water averages 63% of body weight in men and 52% of body weight in women reflects the greater proportion of adipose tissue in women.

Body water is not found in one homogeneous fluid space. Rather, it is distributed among a number of *compartments,* as shown diagrammatically in Figure 1-1. These compartments differ from each other not only in their anatomic locations but also in the composition of their solutes and in their physiologic roles. We'll describe them very briefly.

Intracellular Fluid (Cell Water)

Most of the water in the body—30 to 40% of total body weight—is within cells. The membranes confining this fluid appear to allow the free passage of water, but their vigorous transport mechanisms maintain a solute composition within the cells quite different from that on the outside. They do this by effectively excluding the most common solutes outside the cells—sodium and chloride—and sequestering other ions inside. Thus potassium and magnesium are

1

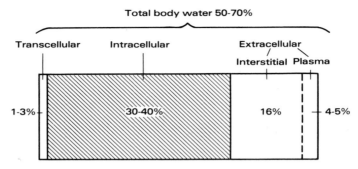

Figure 1-1. Diagrammatic representation of the body fluid compartments. Numbers show the size of each fluid space as a percentage of total body weight. There is considerable variation in these figures because of differences among individuals and among methods used to measure the compartments. We have included the fluid in bone matrix and connective tissue as a part of the interstitial fluid, but some authors prefer to treat them as separate subcompartments because they equilibrate slowly with the rest of the interstitial fluid.

numerically the most important cations dissolved in this cell water, while phosphates and proteins carry most of the anionic charges.

Extracellular Fluid

Extracellular fluid is outside of cells and forms the environment around them. As already noted, the solute composition of this fluid is quite different from that within the cells; sodium is the dominant cation in the extracellular fluid, while chloride and bicarbonate are the major anions. There are two major subdivisions of the extracellular fluid—*plasma water* and *interstitial fluid.*

Plasma water (about 4.5% of body weight) is the water in which blood cells and platelets are suspended and plasma proteins dissolved—the liquid part of the blood, in short. Interstitial fluid (about 16% of body weight) lies outside the blood vessels and surrounds the cells. The only major difference between the solute composition of plasma water and interstitial fluid is the substantial concentration of protein found in plasma water. Since capillaries are quite permeable to the small ions that make up most of the solute in plasma water, the composition of these electrolytes is the same in plasma water and interstitial fluid except for small disparities due to the Donnan effect. The bulk distribution of fluid between plasma water and interstitial fluid is determined by Starling forces. The Donnan effect and Starling forces will both be described later in this chapter.

Transcellular Fluid

Water amounting to 1 to 3% of body weight may be found distributed among a number of pools sequestered by secretory cells from other body fluid compartments. Examples of such fluid collections are the cerebrospinal fluid, the aqueous and vitreous humors of the eye, and the secretions in the gastrointestinal lumen. By literal definition these transcellular fluid pools are a part of the extracellular fluid, since they represent body water not contained within cells. However, they differ from the main body of the extracellular fluid in function and solute composition as well as in location. When we describe the physiological role of the extracellular fluid in later chapters, we shall not consider transcellular water to be a part of it.

Gains, Losses, and Shifts of Fluid

The division of body water into the compartments we have described is of more than academic importance. When fluid balance is upset, the different compartments may or may not be affected in the same way and to the same extent. The possible disturbances are numerous and complex, but a few simple examples here will serve for illustration.

We have already mentioned that water moves in and out of cells freely; this movement occurs passively in response to the concentration of solutes inside and outside of the cells, that is, *osmotic forces*. (See the section on osmolality in this chapter.) Ion pumps in cell membranes, especially sodium-potassium pumps, determine which solutes are kept in cells and which ones are evicted. Let's consider what happens to the volume of intracellular and extracellular fluid when water, sodium chloride or both together are added to the body.

The rectangle on the left side of Figure 1-2 represents the volumes of intracellular and extracellular fluid in a normal person. The rectangles on the right side of the figure show the effect of administering pure water, pure sodium chloride, or both together to this person. To keep our example simple we must assume that the kidneys and thirst mechanism are temporarily asleep and have not yet taken corrective measures.

If pure water is given to our subject, as shown in the top panel on the right,

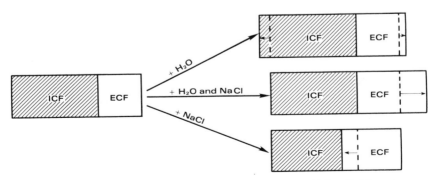

Figure 1-2. Changes in the size of intracellular and extracellular fluid compartments that would be caused by the addition of pure water, pure sodium chloride (NaCl), or both water and NaCl together in isotonic proportions. These figures assume that no compensatory adjustments have occurred.

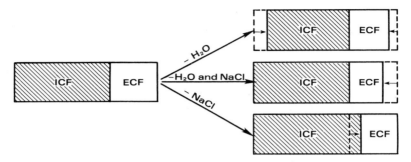

Figure 1-3. Changes in the size of intracellular and extracellular fluid compartments that result from removal of pure water, pure NaCl, or both water and NaCl together in isotonic proportions.

it will be distributed to both intracellular and extracellular fluid in roughly a 2:1 proportion, since the intracellular compartment is twice the size of the extracellular space; both compartments will be diluted.

If pure sodium chloride is given, it will be excluded from cells and confined to the extracellular space. The resulting increase of extracellular solute concentration will cause water to leave the cells, thus enlarging the extracellular space at the expense of intracellular fluid. This is shown by the lowest figure on the right. Though solute has been added to only the extracellular compartment here, osmolality will also rise within the cells because of their water loss.

If both water and sodium chloride are administered in the proportions found in normal plasma, the solute concentration in the body will not change, and there will be no shift of water into or out of cells. This is shown in the middle right-hand figure. Note, however, that all of the administered fluid is now added to the extracellular space alone.

Figure 1-3 depicts the reverse effects—what would happen if pure water, pure sodium chloride, or both together in isotonic proportions could be removed from our subject.

STARLING FORCES

Earlier in the chapter we mentioned that extracellular fluid is distributed between plasma water and interstitial fluid. There is continuous exchange between these compartments. Plasma water is passing through the capillaries into the interstitial space all the time, while an equal amount of interstitial fluid is being restored to the plasma. A disequilibrium between these processes would upset the ratio (normally about 1:4) between plasma volume and the volume of interstitial fluid. Such a disturbance occurs in a number of disease states, but under normal circumstances the losses and gains of plasma water and interstitial fluid are balanced with impressive precision. This is accomplished primarily by the operation of *Starling forces,* named after the English physiologist who suggested their role in 1896.

Stated very simply, Starling forces are hydrostatic pressure, which tends to force fluid out of capillaries, and the colloid osmotic force of dissolved proteins (often referred to as *oncotic pressure*), which tends to bring fluid back into the circulation. At the arterial end of a capillary, the blood pressure in the vessel is high enough to overcome the oncotic force of the plasma proteins. As a result, some plasma water and its small solutes (but not proteins) are forced out into the interstitial space. At the venous end of the capillary, however, the blood pressure has fallen to much lower levels. This allows the osmotic effect of plasma proteins to dominate the situation, with the result that interstitial fluid enters the capillary. A small amount of protein is found normally in the interstitial fluid, but its osmotic effect is usually balanced by the opposing hydrostatic pressure that is also present in the same compartment. These forces are shown diagrammatically in Figure 1-4.

The numbers in Figure 1-4 apply to an ordinary capillary, where the concentration of plasma proteins probably does not change significantly between the arterial and venous ends of the capillary. The same principles can be applied to other vascular beds where the situation is different. In glomerular capillaries, for instance, enough removal of fluid takes place to cause a significant rise in the intravascular protein concentrations. As we shall see, the resulting increase of oncotic pressure has an important effect on both glomerular filtration and the resorption of fluid from renal tubules.

Starling forces can also help us to understand certain disturbances of fluid distribution in the body. For instance, a low concentration of plasma albumin

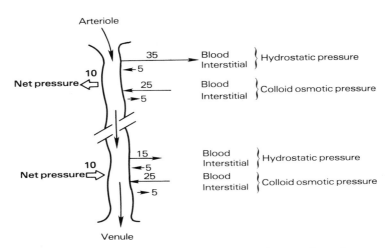

Figure 1-4. Starling forces in a muscle capillary. The figures show the approximate magnitude of each pressure in millimeters mercury.

will lessen oncotic pressure in the capillaries. Unless other factors can compensate for this reduction, there will be a net loss of plasma water into the interstitial space and formation of *edema* (see Chapter 4).

THE DONNAN EQUILIBRIUM

In the preceding section we mentioned the direct osmotic effect exerted by the plasma proteins, which generally cannot pass through capillary walls into the interstitial space. These protein molecules in solution also have an effect on the distribution of small ions across capillary walls.

At the hydrogen-ion concentration found in blood, most plasma protein molecules are anions—that is, they have donated hydrogen ions and now carry a negative charge. Negative charges must be balanced by an equal number of positive charges, of course, and these are provided by small cations such as sodium. This accounts for the fact that there are more small cations (sodium, potassium, and others) in the plasma than small anions (chloride, bicarbonate, and others). To put it in different terms, we might say that some sodium ions are balanced by chloride and bicarbonate, while others are balanced by the anionic proteins.

Figure 1-5 examines what happens (and what doesn't happen) under these circumstances when ions diffuse across a membrane such as a capillary wall. On the left side of each panel we have represented a solution that contains sodium (Na^+), chloride (Cl^-), and protein (Pr^-) in the ionic proportions of 9:4:5. (These numbers don't reflect actual concentrations in the plasma, and they exaggerate the proportion of protein, but they make for easy arithmetic.) Other solutes have been omitted in the interest of simplicity. The solution on the right side of the membrane contains only the solutes that have crossed the membrane from the left side. Our model assumes that the solution in the

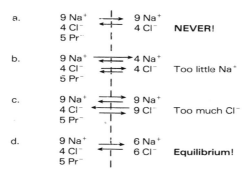

Figure 1-5. Some conceivable (and inconceivable) ways electrolytes might distribute across a semipermeable membrane when an anionic protein (Pr^-) is present on one side. As explained in the text, the situation in panel a is impossible, while the distributions in b and c are unstable. Only d represents an equilibrium.

compartment on the left is continuously replenished, so that its composition remains the same despite diffusion of sodium and chloride ions across the capillary wall.

In the first panel of the figure Na^+ and Cl^- have crossed the membrane, leaving protein behind, until the concentrations of both are equal on both sides. This does not happen, however, because it violates electrochemical principles to have more cations than anions in the compartment on the right side.

Panel b shows the diffusion of Na^+ and Cl^- in equal numbers until the concentration of Cl^- is the same on both sides of the membrane. Chloride is now in equilibrium, but sodium is not, so the tendency for additional Na^+ to cross to the right side makes this an unstable situation.

If Na^+ and Cl^- diffuse together until the concentration of Na^+ is equal on both sides, as shown in panel c, there will be much more Cl^- on the right side of the membrane than the left side. This is not an equilibrium situation due to the tendency of Cl^- to diffuse back to the left.

The chemical compromise that actually occurs is shown in the last panel. At equilibrium the compartment on the right side of the membrane will contain less Na^+ but more Cl^- than the compartment on the left that contains the protein. Donnan demonstrated many years ago that equilibrium is reached when the product of the concentrations of a pair of diffusible ions (in this case Na^+ and Cl^-) is the same on both sides of the membrane. In our example, $9 \times 4 = 6 \times 6$.

A practical effect of this phenomenon is that the concentration of a monovalent cation such as Na^+ is about 5% less in the interstitial fluid than in plasma water, while that of a monovalent anion such as Cl^- is about 5% greater in the interstitial fluid than in plasma. The same relationship holds for the solute content of glomerular filtrate. This difference in solute concentrations on the two sides of a capillary membrane is unimportant for most purposes but must be taken into account when precise measurements and calculations are being made, as in research studies.

An interesting corollary of the Donnan distribution is that the total concentration of *diffusible* ions is slightly greater on the side of the membrane where the nondiffusible protein is located. In terms of the example given in Figure 1-5, $9 + 4 > 6 + 6$. This increase in the total number of diffusible ions augments the direct osmotic effect of the plasma proteins.

WHAT'S OSMOLALITY?

The movements of body water from one compartment to another are often governed by osmotic forces. These forces are determined by the concentrations of solute in the compartments.

When dissolved particles are present in a water solution, the activity or *escaping tendency* of the water molecules in that solution is reduced in proportion to the concentration of dissolved particles. If pure water is placed on one side of a membrane that is permeable only to water molecules, and a solution of any solute in water is placed on the other side, water will escape from the pure-water compartment (where the activity of water is higher) to the compartment containing the solution (Fig. 1-6). If two different solutions are used, water will flow from the less concentrated to the more concentrated one. The ability of a solution to attract water, which reflects the reduced activity of its own water, depends upon its *osmolality*.

Osmolality is simply the concentration of solute molecules in a solvent, expressed as moles (or millimoles) of solute per kilogram of solvent.

You will recall that the molecular weight of any element or compound taken in grams is 1 g molecular weight of that substance, or 1 *mole*. For example, the molecular weight of glucose is 180. Therefore 180 g of glucose is 1 g molecular weight, or 1 mole, of glucose. Since the molecular weight of urea is 60, 1 mole of urea weighs 60 g. One mole of any substance contains the same number of molecules as 1 mole of any other substance: 6.02×10^{23} molecules (Avogadro's number). A millimole is 0.001 mole.

One mole of molecules dissolved in 1 kg of water gives a 1 Osmolal solution.

Examples

180 g glucose in 1 kg of water is a 1 Osmolal solution.
60 g urea in 1 kg of water is a 1 Osmolal solution.

So osmolality is an expression of the concentration of dissolved molecules in a solution, regardless of their nature. If 180 g of glucose and 60 g of urea are dissolved in the same kg of water, we have a solution in which the concentration of glucose is 1 molal and that of urea is 1 molal, but the solution is a 2 Osmolal solution, 1 Osmole contributed by each solute.

When a compound dissociates in solution, osmolality depends upon the number of ions which each molecule produces.

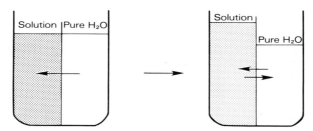

Figure 1-6. Molecules of water will tend to escape from a compartment containing pure water into one that contains water and solute, as shown on the left. The addition of water raises the level of the solute compartment until its hydrostatic pressure equals osmotic pressure. When that point is reached, water transfer across the dividing membrane becomes equal in both directions, as shown in the figure on the right.

Example

One mole of NaCl in 1 kg of water gives a solution that is approximately 2 Osmolal, since the NaCl dissociates almost completely to yield 1 mole of Na^+ ions and 1 mole of Cl^- ions.

Osmolality versus Osmolarity

Osmola*l*ity is the concentration of dissolved particles in solution expressed as moles of solute per *kilogram* of water. Osmola*r*ity is the concentration of dissolved particles in solution expressed as moles of solute per *liter* of the final solution.

If solute is added progressively to 1 kg (1 liter) of pure water, 1 kg of water continues to be present. But the total volume may no longer be 1 liter, since the volume of the solution may increase as solute is added. In concentrated solutions the difference between osmolality and osmolarity may be significant. In the dilute solutions commonly encountered in biology, the difference between osmolality and osmolarity is unimportant, but the use of osmolality is usually preferred for theoretical reasons.

Because body fluids usually have an osmolality less than 1 Osm/kg water, biologists commonly express osmolality in *milli*Osmoles per kilogram of water (1 mOsm = 0.001 Osm). The extracellular fluid of man normally has an osmolality of about 290 mOsm/kg water. Many other species have similar osmolalities.

BIBLIOGRAPHY

The following texts may be consulted for a more detailed presentation of the topics in this chapter:

R. F. Pitts. *Physiology of the kidney and body fluids,* 3rd ed. Chicago: Year Book Medical Publishers, 1974.

B. D. Rose. *Clinical physiology of acid-base and electrolyte disorders.* New York: McGraw-Hill, 1977.

H. Valtin. *Renal function: Mechanisms preserving fluid and solute balance in health.* Boston: Little, Brown, 1973.

Many textbooks of general physiology or biochemistry also include discussions of these subjects.

2
An Overview of Renal Anatomy and Function

THE NEPHRON UNIT

A mammalian kidney is composed primarily of many tiny units called nephrons. In humans there are approximately one million nephrons in each kidney. Each nephron consists of a filtering structure, called the glomerulus, and a long tubule in which the filtrate is partially reabsorbed and modified. It is customary to divide the tubule into several regions: the proximal tubule, the loop of Henle, the distal convoluted tubule, and a collecting duct that is shared by a number of tubules (Fig. 2-1). The distal tubule of each nephron returns past its own glomerulus, having close contact there with the arterioles as they enter and leave the glomerulus.

Nephrons whose glomeruli lie near the surface of the kidney, called *superficial* nephrons, tend to have short loops of Henle. *Juxtamedullary* nephrons, whose glomeruli are found near the junction of the cortex and the medulla (see below), have long loops of Henle that extend deep into the medulla.

GROSS ANATOMY

A normal human kidney averages about 11 to 12 cm in length and 5 to 7 cm in width and weighs about 150 g. If it is sectioned sagittally, different regions can be identified (Fig. 2-2). Beneath the fibrous capsule of the kidney lies the *cortex,* a zone of tissue that includes all of the glomeruli, the convoluted portions of the proximal tubules, the distal convoluted tubules, and the early portions of the collecting ducts. The rest of the active kidney tissue is known as the *medulla,* which is generally divided into the *outer medulla* and the *inner medulla.* The outer medulla, sometimes subdivided into outer and inner stripes, contains the terminal, straight portion (pars recta) of the proximal tubules, loops of Henle from some nephrons and portions of those loops from

11

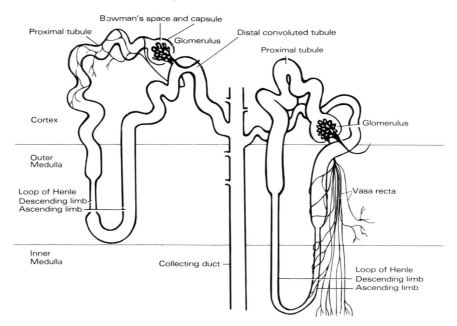

Figure 2-1. Diagrams of two nephrons and their patterns of postglomerular arterial supply. Shown on the left is a superficial cortical nephron; its loop of Henle descends only a short distance into the medulla, and blood leaving the glomerulus supplies tubules in the nearby cortex. The juxtamedullary nephron on the right has a much longer loop of Henle, and its efferent arteriole divides to form the vasa recta which descend deep into the medulla. Venous return, which is not shown, follows a similar pattern.

others, and the middle portion of the collecting ducts. The inner medulla, which is farthest from the cortex, contains thin descending and ascending limbs of loops of Henle from juxtamedullary nephrons, as well as the terminal portions of the collecting ducts (Fig. 2-1). The inner medulla borders on the renal *pelvis,* which is a collecting chamber for the urine as it emerges from the collecting ducts. The loops and ducts of the medulla are arranged into a number of cone-shaped bundles or *pyramids* whose tips project into the renal pelvis and are called *papillae.* (The term *papilla* is also used as a synonym for the entire inner medulla.)

BLOOD SUPPLY

Although the kidneys comprise only 0.5% of the body's weight, they receive a blood flow that is about 20% of the resting cardiac output. Compared with other organs they extract a relatively small percentage of the oxygen available

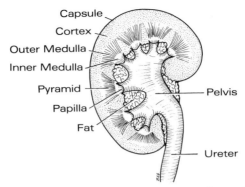

Figure 2-2. Sagittal view of a human kidney showing the major gross anatomical features.

in the blood. This much blood flow would be extravagant for the metabolic needs of the kidneys themselves, but it supports the high rate of filtration that takes place in the kidneys.

Most kidneys have a single renal artery, though the presence of two or more renal arteries is not unusual. The renal artery (or arteries) divides into large anterior and posterior branches and subsequently into segmental or interlobar branches. The latter supply arcuate and interlobular arteries (Fig. 2-3). These are end-arteries without anastomoses, so occlusion of one of these

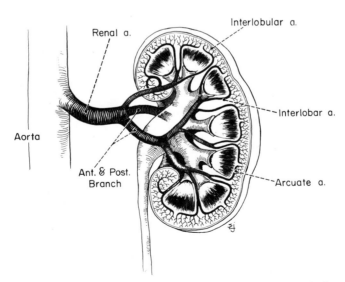

Figure 2-3. The arterial blood supply of a human kidney. Anatomical variations are common, especially in the larger vessels. (From J. Lapides, *Fundamentals of Urology*, Philadelphia, W. B. Saunders Co., 1976. Reproduced with permission.)

vessels causes infarction of the tissue it supplies. The afferent arterioles to the glomeruli come directly from the interlobular arteries. The renal arterial system is short enough and its caliber large enough that blood is delivered to the glomeruli at a mean pressure of about 45 mm Hg, higher than the pressure delivered to most other capillary beds. This feature enables the glomeruli to perform effectively as filters.

Blood leaving the glomeruli in efferent arterioles enters the capillary network surrounding the tubules, usually those in an area close to the glomerulus. (It was once thought that the blood leaving a glomerulus supplies only the corresponding tubule, but this now appears unlikely.) In the case of juxtamedullary glomeruli, however, the efferent arterioles give rise to some long, straight vessels, the *vasa recta,* which supply the renal medulla (Fig. 2-1). The functional significance of these arrangements will be discussed in later chapters.

GLOMERULAR STRUCTURE AND GLOMERULAR FILTRATION

A glomerulus is basically a cluster of specialized capillaries arranged in loops (Fig. 2-4). The capillary walls consist of a basement membrane covered on each side by a single layer of cells (Fig. 2-5). The cells on the inside of the capillary (in contact with the blood) are the endothelial cells. These cells stretch thinly over the basement membrane; by electron microscopy their cytoplasm appears to contain many fenestrations (holes). The epithelial cells

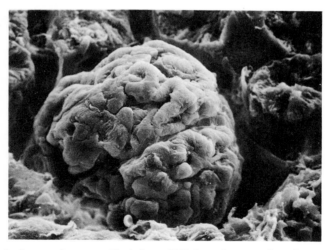

Figure 2-4. A glomerulus magnified about 375 times by scanning electron microscopy. Contours of individual capillary loops are easily seen. (Reproduced with permission from P. M. Burkholder, *Atlas of Human Glomerular Pathology*, New York, Harper & Row, 1974).

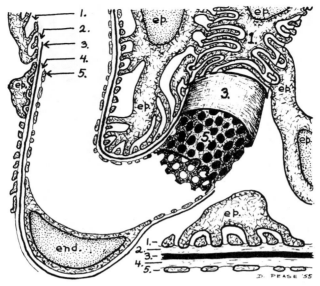

Figure 2-5. This drawing shows the structural components of a glomerular capillary. 1: Foot processes of epithelial cells (ep.); 2–4: basement membrane, which consists of a central dense layer (3) with lighter layers (2 and 4) on each side; 5: fenestrated endothelial cells (end). (From D. C. Pease, *J. Histochem.* 3: 297, 1955. Reproduced with permission.)

sit on the outside of the basement membrane and cover almost all of it with a series of branching projections called foot processes that interdigitate with the foot processes of other epithelial cells (Fig. 2-6). The narrow spaces between the fingerlike foot processes are called slit pores; these slit pores are covered by a very thin membrane.

The route by which water and other molecules from the blood plasma pass through the glomerular capillaries is not completely understood, but it seems likely that they find their way through the fenestrations of the endothelial cells, through the basement membrane itself, and finally through the thin membranes covering the slit pores. We do not know exactly where in these three layers the most important barrier to filtration is located, though most available evidence points to the basement membrane. But the net effect of these structures together is to allow the passage through the capillary wall of only relatively small molecules, while suspended particles and larger molecules, those with a radius of roughly 42Å or more, are kept in the capillary blood. In practical terms this means that red blood cells, white blood cells, platelets, and almost all of the plasma proteins will not be allowed to escape from the glomerular capillaries under normal circumstances.

So the glomerulus can be thought of basically as a very fine sieve or filter. This is an oversimplification, however, since there are no demonstrable

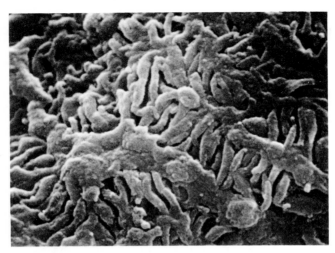

Figure 2-6. A single glomerular capillary loop magnified approximately 7500 times to show how the foot processes of adjacent epithelial cells interdigitate with each other. (Scanning electron micrograph provided by Dr. Peter Burkholder.)

"holes" in the basement membrane and there are factors other than simple molecular size that determine whether a solute will pass through the glomerular barrier. For instance, the shape of a molecule appears to make some difference. And in the case of molecules that are close to the critical size for glomerular filtration, electrical charge influences the ease of passage through the barrier. Some structures of the glomerular wall contain many anionic (negatively charged) proteins; experimental evidence indicates that these repel negatively charged molecules and discourage their filtration, whereas positively charged molecules of the same size pass through easily. Albumin and most other plasma proteins are anions, which may help to explain why they are not filtered under normal circumstances.

As used in common laboratory chemistry, the term *filtration* usually refers to a process that separates particles that are suspended in a liquid medium from those that are in true solution; molecules or ions in true solution pass through the filter, whereas the larger suspended particles do not. It is evident that the process of glomerular filtration goes a step beyond this, since protein molecules that are in true solution and would go through most laboratory filters are prevented from traversing the glomerular barrier. For this reason the term *ultrafiltration* is sometimes applied to the process that takes place in the glomeruli.

Each glomerulus is enveloped by the enlarged initial portion of its own tubule, known as *Bowman's capsule*. This spherical structure surrounds the glomerulus completely and receives its filtrate. The space outside the glomerulus but inside the capsule where glomerular filtrate collects is called *Bowman's space* (Fig. 2-1).

REGIONAL DIFFERENCES IN THE TUBULE

A renal tubule is not a dead pipe. It is lined from Bowman's capsule to the tip of the collecting duct with living cells, each of which has some role in modifying the tubular fluid that comes past it. The responsibilities of these cells vary greatly from one part of the tubule to the next, as will be described in later pages. It is therefore not surprising that some differences in the physical characteristics of the cells can be noted in various regions of the nephron (Fig. 2-7). Only the most striking features will be summarized here.

Cells in the convoluted part of the proximal tubule are distinguished by long, slender structures, or microvilli, which project into the tubular lumen. So numerous are these that in some magnifications they look like the bristles in a brush and are therefore referred to collectively as the *brush border* of the proximal tubule. These microvilli provide a large surface area for exchange between tubular fluid and the cells. The cells themselves are loaded with mitochondria, presumably to support a high level of energy-requiring transport activity.

In the thin segment of Henle's loop we find flat, asthenic-looking cells with few mitochondria. One would not expect from their appearance to find much active transport going on here!

In contrast, the thick ascending limb of Henle's loop is lined with taller, sturdy-looking cells with abundant mitochondria. Compared to the proximal tubule, these cells have rod-shaped mitochondria, and their microvilli appear stubby and less numerous.

The cells of the distal convoluted tubule and collecting duct range from cuboidal to columnar in different regions. They have small microvilli, and the number of mitochondria diminishes in the late part of the distal convoluted tubule and the collecting duct.

An interesting and probably important structure is located in a short segment of the distal tubule where it comes into contact with the arterioles at the vascular entrance to its own glomerulus. The tubular cells here have a distinctive appearance—narrow and tightly packed together—and are referred to as the *macula densa* (dense spot). The cells in the adjacent arterioles at this point are distinctive also and have granules in them that are believed to contain the hormone renin or its precursors. These modified tubular and vascular cells in contact right outside the glomerulus are known together as the *juxtaglomerular apparatus* (JGA).

Sophisticated studies of tubular histology indicate that the tubule has many more distinct regions than the traditional ones we have described; for instance, the proximal and distal tubules could each be subdivided into three

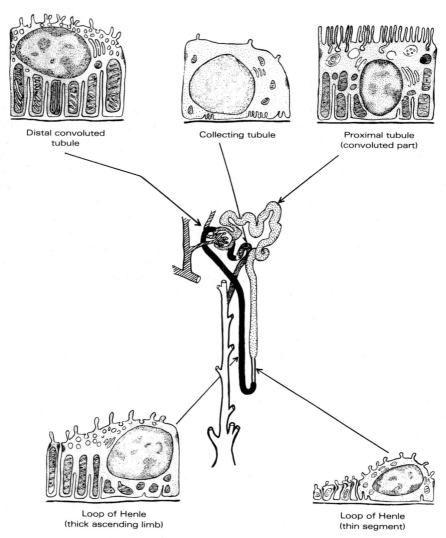

Distal convoluted tubule

Collecting tubule

Proximal tubule (convoluted part)

Loop of Henle (thick ascending limb)

Loop of Henle (thin segment)

Figure 2-7. This drawing shows some of the varying cell types that line different parts of the tubular system. The figure here depicts a superficial nephron that has a short loop of Henle with a greatly attenuated thin segment. The figure labeled "collecting tubule" represents cells in the late distal tubule and early collecting duct, which are very similar. (Adapted from J. Rhodin, *Int. Rev. Cytol.* 7: 506, 1958.)

parts—and maybe more. We shall ignore such subtleties here, however, since they are not essential for a general understanding of renal function.

THROUGH THE NEPHRON BRIEFLY

Dynamics of Glomerular Filtration

The driving force behind glomerular filtration is the hydrostatic pressure ("blood pressure") within the glomerular capillaries, which forces plasma water and its smaller solutes across the filtration barrier. As in other capillaries, this hydrostatic force is opposed by the oncotic force of plasma proteins, which remain within the glomerular capillaries. Filtration is also opposed by the hydrostatic pressure in Bowman's capsule, which is low under normal conditions. So the rate at which glomerular filtrate is formed depends on the balance of these forces as well as on the permeability characteristics of the glomerulus. If the blood pressure in the glomerular capillaries falls below a critical level (perhaps 30 to 35 mm Hg), glomerular filtration will cease completely because the hydrostatic pressure within the capillaries is not sufficient to overcome the opposing forces. And an obstruction downstream in the tubule will tend to raise the pressure in Bowman's capsule and thus reduce the rate of glomerular filtration.

As plasma water is filtered from the glomerular capillaries, the proteins in the capillaries become relatively concentrated, and the resulting increased oncotic pressure at the distal end of a glomerular capillary loop causes a decreased rate or even a cessation of filtration there. Under normal circumstances in humans about 20% of the plasma water that enters the glomeruli is filtered. This figure is known as the *filtration fraction*.

The glomerular filtration rate (GFR) is the total glomerular filtrate formed by all of the glomeruli per unit time. It is usually expressed as milliliters per minute, sometimes as liters per day. In the average-sized man the GFR is about 125 ml/min or 180 liters/day; it is slightly lower for women even when corrected for body size. This awe-inspiring volume made it difficult for early students of renal function to accept the concept of glomerular filtration; it simply did not seem plausible that an individual would filter plasma water far in excess of his own body weight every day. Methods of measuring the GFR and its alterations will be discussed in the next chapter.

Regulation of Glomerular Filtration Rate

As we mentioned earlier, the blood pressure within the glomerular capillaries is the force that causes filtration to occur. We might expect then that the rate of glomerular filtration would vary with the systemic blood pressure, since higher pressure within the capillaries should force more plasma water across the glomeruli. Surprisingly, this does not seem to occur. Animal experiments have demonstrated that the GFR remains relatively constant as blood pressure is raised and lowered over a fairly wide range. This phenomenon, known as *autoregulation of the glomerular filtration rate*, is illustrated in Figure 2-8. Autoregulation is lost at very high blood pressures and also at pressures below a critical level. Obviously filtration cannot occur if hydrostatic pressure in the glomeruli is not sufficient to overcome the oncotic force of the plasma proteins and the hydrostatic pressure in Bowman's capsule.

How does autoregulation happen? It is generally believed that the glomeruli are protected against changes in the systemic blood pressure so that the pressure in the glomerular capillaries remains relatively constant even though systemic blood pressure rises and falls. This may be accomplished by appropriate constriction or relaxation of the afferent arterioles. For instance, if the systemic blood pressure rises, constriction of the afferent arterioles can reduce the pressure actually delivered to the glomeruli. If systemic pressure falls, relaxation of the afferent arterioles can reduce the drop of pressure that normally occurs between the aorta and the glomeruli. It is difficult to find direct proof that these adjustments in the arterioles are in fact taking place, but it is hard to explain autoregulation in any other way. Recent evidence suggests that the efferent arterioles may also have a role in the regulation of GFR.

Autoregulation has been observed to operate in denervated kidneys and even in isolated, artificially perfused kidneys, so it appears not to depend on nervous or hormonal control from outside the kidney. Only a few potent poisons have been found to abolish autoregulation, leading to the belief that

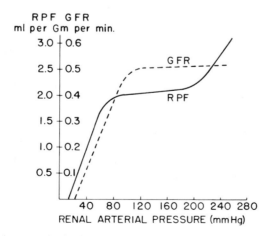

Figure 2-8. Autoregulation of glomerular filtration rate and renal plasma flow in the dog. [Reproduced with permission from R. F. Pitts, *Physiology of the Kidney and Body Fluids*, 3rd ed. Copyright © 1974 by Year Book Medical Publishers, Inc., Chicago. (Adapted from B. Ochwadt, *Prog. Cardiovasc. Dis.* 3: 504, 1961, and redrawn from the work of R. E. Shipley and R. S. Study, *Am. J. Physiol.* 167: 682, 1951.)]

its operation must depend on basic myogenic responses in the afferent and efferent arterioles to changes in systemic blood pressure.

The total renal blood flow appears also to be autoregulated as blood pressure rises and falls (Fig. 2-8). The mechanism is presumably the same as that for autoregulation of GFR.

Although the glomerular filtration rate is not very sensitive to fluctuations in blood pressure and varies relatively little from hour to hour and day to day in normal humans, some conditions will cause it to rise or fall significantly. Probably the most important of these influences is the volume of the extracellular fluid or circulation or both. Expansion of the extracellular fluid volume is likely to be accompanied by an increase in the GFR, and an actual or perceived depletion of the extracellular fluid or circulatory volume may cause marked reduction of the GFR. The latter may occur without any impressive fall of the systemic blood pressure, so it appears that blood flow to the kidneys (as well as to a number of other organs) may be sacrificed at times to permit the maintenance of adequate blood pressure to the heart, lungs, and brain. (It follows that the presence of a normal systemic blood pressure does not prove that there is good blood flow in the kidneys.)

In stressful situations such as severe exertion, GFR and renal blood flow may also be curtailed. The mechanism of this reduction is probably arteriolar constriction in response to neurogenic and possibly hormonal messages.

Action in the Proximal Tubules

Our knowledge of what happens in the proximal tubules, or in any specific part of the tubular system for that matter, is based primarily on micropuncture studies of rats, dogs and monkeys. We assume that human kidneys are quite similar to those of our mammalian relatives.

An enormous amount of plasma water enters the tubules as glomerular filtrate each day. Only about 1% of that water, with its solute content markedly altered, reaches the renal pelvis as urine. Of the many modifications that must take place to change plasma water to urine, the most numerous and quantitatively most important ones take place in the proximal tubules.

By the time the tubular fluid reaches the end of the proximal tubules, about 70% of its sodium, almost that much of its chloride, 80 to 90% of its bicarbonate and about 70% of its water have been reabsorbed into the circulation. The resorption of sodium and bicarbonate appears to involve active processes (see Chapters 5 and 7), while that of chloride appears to be passive in the proximal tubule. Since the sodium, chloride, and bicarbonate ions together comprise over 90% of the solute particles in plasma water, it is evident that most of the solute in plasma water gets removed in the proximal tubules. This would leave the tubular fluid very hypo-osmotic were it not for the fact that the proximal tubules are freely permeable to water. Because of this permeability, water is reabsorbed passively by osmotic forces in close parallel with the active resorption of sodium. So the fluid in the proximal tubules remains isotonic with plasma water, and the sodium concentration at the end of the proximal tubules is about the same as at the beginning, because sodium and water have left the tubules in the same proportions. This also reduces the work the proximal tubules must do to reabsorb all that sodium, since they do not have to move it against a significant gradient.

Many other resorptive processes also take place in the proximal tubule. In addition to sodium, chloride, and bicarbonate, glomerular filtrate contains many other ions and small molecules whose loss in the urine would be distinctly disadvantageous. These losses are prevented under normal circumstances by resorption that takes place largely in the proximal tubules. For instance, most of the filtered potassium, calcium, and magnesium are reabsorbed proximally, though a portion of these ions must also be excreted in the urine (especially in the case of potassium) if excessive accumulation in the body is to be avoided. Some other essential small solutes, such as glucose and amino acids, are removed from the tubular fluid almost completely under normal circumstances by active transport mechanisms in the proximal tubules.

The resorption of glucose from proximal tubular fluid provides an example of these active transport mechanisms. It appears that a specific carrier protein on the luminal border of the proximal tubular cells combines with glucose and carries it into the cells, from which it finds its way back into the circulation. We know that this is an active (energy-requiring) process because glucose is moved against a concentration gradient. Like most other active transport arrangements, this system has a limited capacity and can be saturated if too much glucose appears in the tubular fluid; under such circumstances the glucose that cannot be reabsorbed passes into the more distal parts of the tubular system and usually reaches the urine eventually. We say then that the *threshold* for glucose resorption has been exceeded. If the glomerular filtration rate remains constant, variations in the amount of glucose delivered to the tubules will depend on the concentration of glucose in plasma water (and thus in the glomerular filtrate).

Figure 2-9 shows the findings from an experiment in which the plasma glucose concentration of a subject was raised progressively while GFR and urinary glucose content were followed. Assuming a fairly stable rate of glomerular filtration in this normal subject, we know that the amount of glucose filtered by glomeruli rises in a linear fashion as plasma glucose rises. Initially all filtered glucose is reabsorbed. When the threshold level is reached, resorption can increase no further; additional filtered glucose above that level is excreted in the urine. These relationships are shown in the figure. You will note that there is some curvature or *splay* in the lines for resorption and excretion near the threshold level of plasma glucose. This may mean that not all nephrons have exactly the same balance between filtering and resorptive capacity, so that not all tubules get saturated simultaneously. It may also mean that the carrier molecules begin to allow the escape of some glucose in the tubular fluid before they have reached the absolute limit of their transporting

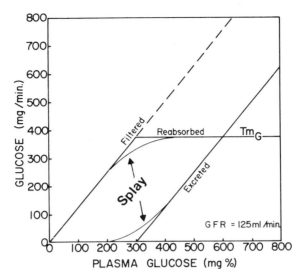

Figure 2-9. Glucose titration curves in normal man, showing the amount of glucose filtered by glomeruli, reabsorbed by tubules, and excreted in the urine as the plasma glucose concentration is raised progressively. Tm_G = transport maximum for glucose. (Slightly modified from R. F. Pitts, *Physiology of the Kidney and Body Fluids*, 3rd ed., Chicago, Year Book Medical Publishers, 1974.)

capacity—sometimes called the *transport maximum* for glucose or simply *Tm glucose.*

We know that glucose resorption is really more complicated than this. The Tm glucose is not fixed; it is influenced by other factors such as the rate of sodium resorption and the volume of the extracellular fluid. But the general concept is still valid that glucose is completely reabsorbed unless the tubular capacity to reabsorb it is exceeded. When the tubular capacity is exceeded because of high plasma glucose levels, as happens frequently in patients with diabetes mellitus, the resulting glucosuria is simply an overflow phenomenon that does not imply renal dysfunction. The presence of glucose in the urine when plasma levels of glucose are not increased is much less common. This so-called *renal glucosuria* suggests a tubular disorder.

Like glucose, amino acids are almost completely reabsorbed from the tubular fluid by active transport under normal circumstances. And similar to glucose, their appearance in the urine may result from high plasma levels that overflow resorptive mechanisms or from tubular dysfunction. Since a number of different transport systems are involved in the resorption of the various amino acids, different patterns of aminoaciduria may occur as a result of tubular dysfunction, depending on the defective transport system.

Phosphorus is a vital constituent of the body but also a waste product, since most diets contain phosphorus in excess of actual needs. The kidneys must dispose of the extra phosphorus, largely in the form of phosphate ions, while retaining enough phosphorus to maintain proper phosphate levels in body fluids. Under normal circumstances about 85% of the phosphate in glomerular filtrate is reabsorbed in the proximal tubules, while about 15% appears in the urine. The resorption of phosphorus can be regulated in response to needs, however. The major mechanism for this regulation under most circumstances involves parathyroid hormone, which has an inhibitory effect on the tubular resorption of phosphate. If serum phosphate begins to increase, it tends to decrease the concentration of ionized calcium. The decrease in ionized calcium then stimulates the secretion of parathyroid hormone, which decreases tubular resorption of phosphate and allows more phosphorus to be excreted in the urine. This lowers serum phosphate, and homeostasis is restored. Conversely, a decrease of serum phosphorus typically results in decreased urinary excretion of phosphate.

Uric acid is also reabsorbed in the proximal tubule, though it's hard to understand why, since it seems to have no role in the body except as a waste product which can cause trouble when present in excess. (Fortunately, uric acid is also secreted by the proximal tubule.)

Tubular Secretion

It is often said that urine formation involves three processes: filtration, resorption, and secretion. We have already discussed filtration and resorption. Secretion is the movement of substances in a direction opposite to that of resorption, that is, from the peritubular circulation into the tubular fluid. In the proximal tubule, secretion seems to involve carrier systems that transport actively against gradients and that can be saturated.

Three secretory carrier systems have been identified in the proximal tubule. One transports a group of compounds, many of which are weak organic acids; the group includes penicillin, chlorothiazide, phenol red, p-aminohippurate (PAH), some radiographic contrast agents, and others. Another carrier system secretes a group of organic bases such as histamine, thiamine, choline, and guanidine. Curiously, the third carrier system appears to secrete only ethylenediaminetetraacetate (EDTA); one wonders if it may not have some other function yet to be discovered.

Tubular secretion in the proximal tubule has several important implications and applications:

1. Tubular secretion of some drugs may remove them from the body fluids faster than if they were eliminated by glomerular filtration alone. This is true, for instance, for penicillin, which has a renal clearance higher than the glomerular filtration rate. This can occur because virtually all of the renal blood flow passes through the capillary network around the tubules. In contrast, only about 20% of the renal plasma flow is filtered through the glomerular capillary walls.

2. Compounds that are secreted by the same carrier system may compete with each other. For instance, PAH interferes with the secretion of penicillin.
3. The efficient tubular secretion of PAH makes it possible to use the clearance of PAH as a measure of renal plasma flow; the rationale for this is presented in the next chapter.

It will be evident by this time that the proximal tubule is the workhorse of the nephron; in the variety of functions performed and the volume of material transported it has no equal. But at the end of the proximal tubule we still find a large volume of isotonic tubular fluid that needs a great deal of refinement in order to become respectable urine. The finishing touches are applied in the remainder of the nephron.

The Loop of Henle

The loop of Henle makes possible the formation of a concentrated urine and also contributes to the formation of dilute urine. How this is accomplished is the subject of Chapter 6. Suffice it to say here that there is further resorption of tubular fluid—perhaps 5 to 15% of the glomerular filtrate—and further net resorption of chloride and sodium in the loop of Henle. The fluid that emerges from the loop is always hypotonic, regardless of whether concentrated or dilute urine is being produced.

Distal Convoluted Tubule and Collecting Duct

The distal convoluted tubule and the collecting duct can be considered together because they perform many of the same functions. Furthermore, some histologic and physiological studies indicate that the last part of the distal tubule is very similar to the first part of the collecting duct, suggesting that the usual dividing line between them is an artificial one.

From the ascending limb of Henle's loop the distal tubule receives about 15 to 20% of the water in the original glomerular filtrate and 5 to 10% of the sodium originally filtered. Since only about 1% of the filtered water and 0.5% of the filtered sodium usually appear in the final urine, it is evident that significant resorption of water and sodium must be taking place in the distal tubule or collecting duct or both. Sodium resorption in this portion of the nephron takes place against a steep concentration gradient and is stimulated, at least in some areas, by the hormone aldosterone. Under appropriate circumstances almost all sodium can be removed from the tubular fluid.

Resorption of water in the distal tubule and collecting duct is passive in response to osmotic forces, as in the proximal tubule. But unlike the proximal tubule, the distal tubule and collecting duct are not freely permeable to water at all times. Their permeability is regulated by the presence or absence of vasopressin, the antidiuretic hormone. Variations in membrane permeability caused by this hormone determine how much water actually leaves the tubular fluid in response to osmotic forces and whether the urine will consequently be concentrated or dilute. In this respect, at least, there is a clear separation between the functions of the distal tubule and the collecting duct: The distal tubule can probably raise the osmolality of the tubular fluid to a level isotonic with plasma, but only the collecting duct can produce hypertonic tubular fluid, for reasons that will be made clear in Chapter 6.

Although the proximal tubule processes and reabsorbs far more sodium and water than the distal tubule and collecting duct, the latter segments appear to have the last word, since they regulate the amount of sodium and water that are actually discarded in the urine.

Another important function of the distal convoluted tubule/collecting duct is the secretion of hydrogen ions. Total hydrogen-ion secretion here is far less than in the proximal tubule. But hydrogen-ion secretion in the proximal tubule is used up almost entirely in reabsorbing filtered bicarbonate, and the pH of the tubular fluid changes very little. In contrast, hydrogen-ion secretion in the distal tubule or collecting duct can produce a marked fall in the pH of the tubular fluid, since almost no bicarbonate remains at this point. Again the distal tubule and collecting duct have the last word, regulating the net acid excretion of the kidney to preserve acid-base homeostasis in the body. This process is treated in more detail in Chapter 7.

Renal excretion of the important potassium ion is also regulated in the distal tubule and collecting duct. Although much of the potassium in the glomerular filtrate has been reabsorbed by the time the tubular fluid reaches the distal nephron, it is secretion of potassium ions into the lumen of the distal tubule and collecting duct that determines the amount of potassium eliminated from the body. Under some circumstances the amount of potassium in the urine may exceed the amount that was filtered—convincing proof of a secretory process. The factors regulating potassium secretion are discussed in Chapter 8.

BIBLIOGRAPHY

B. M. Brenner and R. Beeuwkes III. The renal circulations. *Hosp. Prac.* 13: 35–46, July 1978.

> *Though this review focuses on microvascular arrangements in the kidney, it touches upon several areas of renal physiology, including the dynamics of glomerular filtration and material that is presented in Chapters 5 and 6.*

B. M. Brenner, T. H. Hostetter, and H. D. Humes. Glomerular permselectivity: Barrier function based on discrimination of molecular size and charge. *Am. J. Physiol.* 234: F455–F460, 1978.

> *Discussion of factors that determine what passes through the glomerulus, with review of some supporting evidence.*

E. M. Renkin and R. R. Robinson. Glomerular filtration. *N. Engl. J. Med.* 290: 785–792, 1974.

Discussion of glomerular permeability and the determinants, measurement, and clinical implications of changes in glomerular filtration rate.

C. Tisher. Functional anatomy of the kidney. *Hosp. Prac.* 13: 53–65, May 1978.

A detailed but readable description, with numerous photomicrographs of the cells found in different parts of the nephron, together with some discussion of functional correlates. The author provides considerable information about the histologic subdivisions of various tubular segments that were largely ignored in this chapter.

M. A. Venkatashalam and H. Rennke. The structural and molecular basis of glomerular filtration. *Circ. Res.* 43: 337–347, 1978.

Describes the factors that may explain the selective permeability of the glomerulus.

3
Measurement of Glomerular Filtration Rate; Use of the Clearance Concept

Urine formation begins with glomerular filtration and cannot take place without it. As we have seen, the glomeruli of a normal person filter an enormous quantity of fluid each day. This became apparent when methods were developed to calculate the glomerular filtration rate (GFR)—the rate at which plasma water is being sieved by all of an individual's glomeruli together. The measurement of GFR now has many applications in research and is useful in clinical medicine as well. When diseases cause the destruction of renal tissue, the decrease of glomerular filtration rate usually parallels the loss of tissue and of other renal functions, so measurements or estimates of the GFR are commonly used as indicators of overall renal function. Because the determination of GFR has so many important applications, every student of the kidney should understand the concepts and the simple calculations employed.

First, let's consider the characteristics of inulin, which made possible the measurement of GFR.

1. Inulin is an inert polymer of fructose with a molecular weight of about 5000 and a molecular radius of about 15 Å. It is therefore a small enough molecular to be filtered "freely" with plasma water by the glomeruli— meaning that it is not held back by the glomerular filtration barrier.

2. Inulin is not bound to plasma proteins. Therefore all of the inulin in plasma is available for filtration.

It follows from 1 and 2 that the concentration of inulin in glomerular filtrate is the same as its concentration in plasma water. Thus a measurement of plasma inulin gives us its concentration in Bowman's capsule also. Though it is very difficult to collect fluid from Bowman's capsule, it is easy to get plasma for analysis.

3. The renal tubules ignore inulin. They do not reabsorb it from the fluid in the tubules, nor do they add any inulin to the tubular fluid. Inulin passes from Bowman's capsule to the final urine unmolested, though its concentration changes as water is resorbed (Fig. 3-1). So all the inulin that was filtered by the glomeruli gets into the final urine, and all the inulin in the urine got there by glomerular filtration. On the basis of these facts we can set up a simple equation:

(A) Inulin filtered (mg/min) = inulin reaching the urine (mg/min)

The total inulin filtered per minute is equal to the glomerular filtration rate (ml/min) times the concentration of inulin in the glomerular filtrate. As already explained, the concentration of inulin in the glomerular filtrate is equal to its concentration in the plasma (P_{IN}). So:

(B) Inulin filtered (mg/min) = GFR (ml/min) $\times$ P_{IN} (mg/ml)

The inulin reaching the urine per minute equals the concentration of inulin in urine (U_{IN}) multiplied by the rate of urine flow (V) in milliliters per minute:

(C) Inulin reaching the urine (mg/min) = U_{IN} (mg/ml) $\times$ V (ml/min)

So substituting (B) and (C) in (A), we have

$$\text{GFR (ml/min)} \times P_{IN} = U_{IN} \times V \text{ (ml/min)}$$

or

$$\text{GFR (ml/min)} = \frac{U_{IN} \times V \text{ (ml/min)}}{P_{IN}}$$

Since all the factors on the right side of the last equation are measurable, we can obtain enough data to calculate the GFR. This measure of GFR with the use of inulin is also known as the inulin *clearance,* since it tells us how many milliliters of plasma could have been completely cleared of inulin each minute—if continuous mixing of plasma were not taking place, of course.

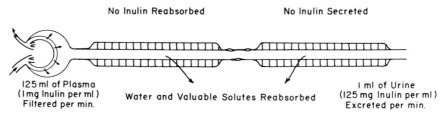

No Inulin Reabsorbed   No Inulin Secreted

125 ml of Plasma
(1 mg Inulin per ml)
Filtered per min.   Water and Valuable Solutes Reabsorbed   1 ml of Urine
(125 mg Inulin per ml)
Excreted per min.

Figure 3-1. Diagram illustrating the fact that the amount of inulin excreted is equal to the amount filtered by the glomeruli, though the concentration of inulin changes markedly during passage through the tubules. (Reproduced with permission from R. F. Pitts, *Physiology of the Kidney and Body Fluids*, 3rd ed. Copyright © 1974 by Year Book Medical Publishers, Inc., Chicago.)

The renal clearance (C) of any other substance (z) can be measured using the same formula:

$$C_z(ml/min) = \frac{U_z \times V \ (ml/min)}{P_z}$$

where U_z is the concentration of z in urine, P_z is the concentration of z in plasma, and V is the rate of urine flow.

As in the case of inulin, this clearance value tells us how many milliliters of plasma could be completely cleared of substance z each minute by the kidneys. Or to state the same idea a bit differently, C_z is a measure of how many milliliters of plasma would be needed each minute to provide the amount of z being excreted in the urine.

Although the clearance of any substance that is excreted by the kidneys can be measured using the same formula we used for inulin clearance, such clearances are equal to the GFR only in the case of inulin and one or two other compounds. This is because other substances lack the described properties of inulin. For example, if a substance is either reabsorbed or secreted by the renal tubules, the assumptions that allowed us to write equation (A) are no longer valid. Nevertheless, clearance measurements for other compounds, when compared with the clearance of inulin, can yield valuable information about their fate in the tubules. For instance, a substance that is filtered and partially reabsorbed will have a clearance lower than that of inulin.

Although inulin is the standard for the measurement of GFR, determination of its clearance is cumbersome. Since it does not occur naturally in the body, it must be infused intravenously until a stable concentration in the plasma is achieved. This is necessary in order that one or two measurements of plasma inulin will accurately reflect the inulin concentration in glomerular filtrate over the entire time required for a clearance measurement. The laboratory determination of inulin concentrations is also rather burdensome. For these reasons simpler methods of measuring GFR have been sought. The clearance of iothalamate is essentially identical to that of inulin and hence a good measure of GFR. Because iothalamate can be tagged with ^{131}I, its concentrations can be measured by counting radioactivity, thus avoiding cumbersome laboratory analyses—but iothalamate must still be infused intravenously.

The use of the creatinine clearance has provided an acceptable compromise between convenience and accuracy in clinical situations. Creatinine, a product of muscle metabolism, is produced in the body at a rate that is remarkably constant for each person. It is a small molecule that is not bound to plasma proteins and filters easily through the glomeruli. Creatinine is excreted in humans primarily by glomerular filtration, and its plasma level changes very little when renal function is stable. This naturally occurring plasma level obviates the need to employ intravenous infusions. Because some creatinine is secreted by the renal tubules in man, creatinine clearances are higher than inulin clearances, but the error is not clinically important unless severe renal failure is present. For these reasons the creatinine clearance is often used in clinical settings to provide an approximate measure of GFR:

$$C_{cr} = \frac{U_{cr} \times V\ (ml/min)}{P_{cr}} \cong GFR$$

Before we leave the equation for creatinine clearance, we should call attention to some other useful information available from these figures. The ratio U_{cr}/P_{cr} is a reflection of how much of the glomerular filtrate was reabsorbed in the tubules (if we disregard tubular secretion and assume that all the creatinine in the urine got there by filtration). For instance, if U_{cr} is 100 times P_{cr}, the creatinine in the urine must be concentrated in only 1/100 of the fluid volume of the original glomerular filtrate. That tells us that 99% of the water in glomerular filtrate is being reabsorbed and 1% is reaching the urine.

If the urine has been collected for 24 hours, the urine concentration of creatinine can be multiplied by the *total* urine volume, to give the total daily creatinine excretion:

$$U_{cr}\ (mg/ml) \times V\ (ml/day) = \text{creatinine excretion (mg/day)}$$

(Be careful of the units in this calculation. U_{cr} is often reported by the laboratory as mg/*dl*, which must be converted to mg/ml for this equation.) Since total daily creatinine excretion is fairly constant for each person, this figure can tell us if the urine collection is complete, provided that we know the usual creatinine output of this individual.

INDIRECT ESTIMATION OF GFR

Under stable conditions of renal function, creatinine enters the blood from muscle metabolism at a constant rate and is removed by the kidneys at the same constant rate. In other words, the number of milligrams of creatinine produced per minute is equal to the number of milligrams of creatinine excreted per minute. And if we assume that all creatinine is excreted by glomerular filtration (ignoring the small component of tubular secretion), the number of milligrams of creatine excreted per minute equals the glomerular filtration rate multiplied by the concentration of creatinine in the plasma water (P_{cr}) being filtered:

$$\text{Creatinine excreted (mg/min)} = GFR\ (ml/min) \times P_{cr}\ (mg/ml)$$

If the GFR remains fairly constant, the plasma creatinine concentration will also remain constant at a level such that the amount of creatinine filtered and excreted each minute is equal to the creatinine production in the body.

Let's see what happens when glomerular filtration is reduced, as happens in a number of renal diseases that destroy glomeruli. A person with a normal GFR is represented in the first panel of Figure 3-2 by eight glomeruli. This individual has a plasma creatinine concentration of 1 mg/dl, which is also the

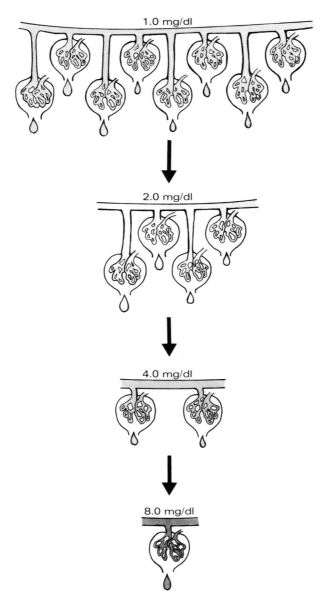

Figure 3-2. The relationship of plasma creatinine concentration (shown above the blood vessel in each panel) to progressive loss of nephrons. The text explains why creatinine concentration rises as nephrons are lost.

concentration of creatinine in each drop of glomerular filtrate. Now suppose that this person loses one-half of his glomeruli and the GFR is cut in half, as represented by the four glomeruli in the next panel. The immediate effect is that the amount of creatinine filtered and excreted (GFR × P_{cr}) will be cut in half. Creatinine continues to be produced by muscle tissues at an unchanged rate, however, and will now accumulate in the body, since excretion has been reduced. As creatinine accumulates, the plasma concentration of creatinine (P_{cr}) rises. And as P_{cr} rises, more creatinine is contained in each drop of glomerular filtrate. When the plasma creatinine concentration reaches 2 mg/dl, each drop of glomerular filtrate will contain twice as much creatinine as previously. This means that the total amount of creatinine filtered and excreted will now be the same as it was originally, even though only half as many drops of filtrate are being formed. At this point the excretion rate of creatinine will again equal the production rate, creatinine will not continue to accumulate, and the plasma creatinine concentration will stabilize at 2 mg/dl. A new steady state has been achieved.

The last two panels of Figure 3-2 represent two further 50% reductions of glomerular filtration rate; each is accompanied by a doubling of the plasma creatinine concentration. This rise of plasma creatinine concentration makes it possible in each case to achieve a new steady state in which creatinine excretion equals creatinine production even though GFR has been drastically reduced. And it explains a fact that at first appears to defy common sense— that an individual with severely impaired renal function (reduced GFR) can and usually does excrete as much total creatinine each day as he did when his kidney function was normal. Of course, this can be achieved only because the plasma creatinine is elevated to many times its normal concentration.

The simple inverse relationship between GFR (represented as creatinine clearance) and the plasma creatinine level is shown graphically in Figure 3-3. If one factor doubles (multiplied by 2), the other is reduced by one-half (muliplied by $\frac{1}{2}$); if one factor increases to $\frac{3}{2}$ of its original value, the other will be reduced to $\frac{2}{3}$ of its original value, and so forth.

Example

A patient with renal disease has a creatinine clearance of 60 ml/min and plasma creatinine = 2 mg/dl. Several months later the plasma creatinine has risen to 3 mg/dl. What is the creatinine clearance now?

Answer

40 ml/min.

It is easy to see from the curve in Figure 3-3 that at low levels of creatinine clearance a small further reduction in clearance will cause the plasma creatinine to rise sharply. To put this in different terms, a small loss of renal function will have little chemical impact on a previously normal person, but it may make an important difference to a patient whose renal function is already poor.

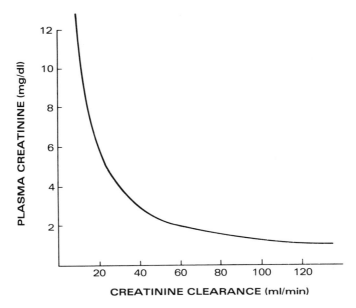

Figure 3-3. The relationship of plasma creatinine to creatinine clearance in a typical person, assuming constant production of creatinine. The points would be slightly different for another person with a different rate of creatinine production, but the curve would have the same shape.

Once the relationship between creatinine clearance and plasma creatinine has been established for an individual, measurement of the plasma creatinine alone enables one to make a reasonable estimate of the creatinine clearance. So the plasma creatinine (actually measured as *serum* creatinine by most laboratories) is widely used by clinicians to follow changes in the renal function of their patients. Compared with measurement of the creatinine clearance, plasma creatinine is a somewhat more dependable test, since it does not involve the collection of a timed urine specimen—the source of much error in clearance determinations. And plasma creatinine is also a less expensive test than the creatinine clearance, since it involves one chemical determination instead of two.

Then why should one ever determine the creatinine clearance if the measurement of plasma creatinine alone is cheaper and more dependable? The main reason is that creatinine production, though quite constant for each person, varies considerably among persons (even among those of the same sex and comparable size). Inequalities in muscle mass or development may account for the differences. Table 3-1 gives some illustrative figures for two male students whom we'll call Fauntleroy and Hercules.

Although Fauntleroy and Hercules have the same glomerular filtration rate (measured as creatinine clearance), Hercules has a higher plasma creatinine

Table 3-1. How creatinine production influences plasma creatinine.

	Weight (kg)	Creatinine Clearance (ml/min)	Daily Creatinine Production (mg/day)	Plasma Creatinine (mg/dl)
Fauntleroy	80	125	1260	0.7
Hercules	80	125	2520	1.4

concentration because his daily production of creatinine is much greater. If we had no information other than the plasma creatinine levels, we might conclude incorrectly that Fauntleroy has a better GFR than Hercules.

At any other level of GFR, Hercules' higher rate of creatinine production will cause him to have higher plasma creatinine values than Fauntleroy. For instance, if both men were to lose all but 10% of their kidney function, Hercules would have a plasma creatinine of about 14 mg/dl, while Fauntleroy's plasma creatinine would be only 7 mg/dl. In the absence of other information, Hercules would appear to have more advanced renal failure than Fauntleroy, but measurement of their creatinine clearances would reveal the true state of things.

The creatinine clearance is also quite useful when the glomerular filtration rate is changing rapidly over a period of hours or a few days. As we have already seen, plasma creatinine concentration reaches a balance point with each level of creatinine clearance (Figs. 3-2 and 3-3). But it takes some time for this to happen, and in acute situations the plasma creatinine may not have caught up with a rapidly changing GFR. For instance, if a previously normal person suddenly loses almost all kidney function, his plasma creatinine level the next day will be only moderately elevated; it may take a week for plasma creatinine to accumulate to a level that reflects the degree of renal impairment. But the creatinine clearance will show a profound fall right away.

Urea Clearance and Plasma Urea

In man and most other mammals, urea is the major waste product of nitrogen metabolism. Quantitatively, at least, its elimination is one of the major responsibilities of the kidneys. Urea enters the tubular fluid in the glomerular filtrate, but much of the filtered urea diffuses back into the circulation as the fluid passes through the tubules. Elevation of the urea concentration in the blood is the most conspicuous chemical abnormality that results from kidney failure.

The clearance of urea can be measured using the same clearance formula we used for unulin and creatinine. If urea clearance is plotted against its plasma concentration, we get the same relationship and the same type of curve as we did (Fig. 3-3) for creatinine clearance and plasma creatinine; that is, as one variable rises, the other decreases by the same proportion. With a rationale similar to that for the use of creatinine clearance and plasma creatinine determinations, urea clearances and blood urea have been used as indicators of glomerular filtration rate.*

However, urea clearances and blood urea nitrogen levels are less satisfactory than the corresponding creatinine measurements for several reasons. First, urea clearance is only 60 to 40% of the true GFR because 40 to 60% of the urea filtered by the glomeruli is reabsorbed passively in the tubules. If the proportion of tubular resorption were constant, we could correct for it, but it varies with the rate of urine flow (which is virtually independent of GFR, as we will see in another chapter): Less urea is reabsorbed at high rates of urine flow. There are formulas that provide an approximate correction for the rate of urine flow, but why bother if you can get a creatinine clearance instead?

Use of the BUN as an indirect measure of GFR has even more problems. Changes in the rate of urine flow that have little relation to GFR will influence the blood urea level because, as we have just noted, they affect urea clearance. Furthermore, unlike the production of creatinine, the rate of urea production in the body is not constant; it may be increased by a high protein intake, gastrointestinal bleeding, or the administration of corticosteroid hormones. Any of these influences can raise the blood urea to abnormally high levels even though renal function is normal. In short, the BUN is not a conclusive test of anything because it reflects a number of factors. Even so, glomerular filtration is probably the most important of those factors, and renal dysfunction must be considered among other possible explanations for an elevated BUN. And a BUN that is very high, not just moderately elevated, almost always indicates a major reduction of the glomerular filtration rate.

MEASUREMENT OF RENAL PLASMA FLOW

In the preceding chapter we mentioned briefly that the clearance of p-aminohippurate (PAH) can be used to measure renal plasma flow:

$$C_{PAH} \cong RPF$$

This is another use of the clearance concept. This application depends upon the ability of the renal tubules to remove PAH from the blood plasma very efficiently—so efficiently, in fact, that virtually all PAH can be removed from the plasma under some circumstances in a single pass through the kidney.

The rationale is as follows: The amount of PAH that appears in the urine

*Several ways of describing blood urea concentrations have evolved and may be confusing. Urea can be measured in whole blood, plasma, or serum—it doesn't seem to make much difference. Even though the determination is commonly performed now on serum, it is often still described as *blood urea nitrogen* or simply BUN. American laboratories usually express their results in terms of the milligrams of nitrogen present as urea, as these terms imply. But laboratories in the United Kingdom often report the total milligrams of urea present. So Englishmen produce higher numbers than Americans, since 60 mg of urea contains only 28 mg of nitrogen.

each minute must equal the amount of PAH removed from the plasma each minute:

(D) PAH in urine (mg/min) = PAH removed from plasma (mg/min)

The amount of PAH in the urine per minute is obtained by multiplying the urinary concentration of PAH (U_{PAH}) by the urine volume (V) per minute:

(E) PAH in urine (mg/min) = U_{PAH} (mg/ml) × V (ml/min)

The amount of PAH removed from the plasma each minute is obtained by multiplying the renal plasma flow by the difference between the concentration of PAH in the renal artery (A_{PAH}) and its concentration in the renal vein (V_{PAH}):

$$\text{(F) PAH removed from plasma (mg/min)} = \text{RPF (ml/min)} \times (A_{PAH} - V_{PAH}) \text{ (mg/ml)}$$

Substituting (E) and (F) into (D), we have

$$U_{PAH} \times V = RPF \times (A_{PAH} - V_{PAH})$$

Direct measurements have shown that at low plasma concentrations of PAH, the PAH concentration in renal venous plasma (V_{PAH}) is essentially zero. So V_{PAH} can be eliminated from the preceding equation:

$$U_{PAH} \times V = RPF \times A_{PAH}$$

or

$$RPF = \frac{U_{PAH} \times V}{A_{PAH}}$$

Since PAH is not extracted by other tissues, arterial PAH is equal to the PAH concentration in peripheral venous plasma (P_{PAH}), so

$$RPF = \frac{U_{PAH} \times V}{P_{PAH}}$$

You will recognize that this is the standard clearance equation (in this case an expression for PAH clearance).

Since PAH is a substance foreign to the body, it must be infused at a steady rate (like inulin) during a clearance determination. We must remember that C_{PAH} = RPF only at low plasma levels of PAH. At higher plasma levels the tubular secretory capacity for PAH (T_m PAH) is exceeded, and PAH is no longer removed completely from the renal plasma. It is also true that a small fraction of renal blood flow passes through tissues that cannot extract PAH; so to this extent the assumption that there is no PAH left in the renal venous blood is an oversimplification, and C_{PAH} slightly underestimates the true renal plasma flow. Despite these limitations, this method of measuring RPF without having to collect blood from the renal vein has been useful in many studies of renal function. Renal plasma flow can be converted to renal blood flow by applying a correction factor for the volume of red cells in whole blood.

BIBLIOGRAPHY

J. P. Kassirer. Clinical evaluation of kidney function—Glomerular function. *N. Engl. J. Med.* 285: 385–389, 1971.

Other discussions of the material in this chapter may be found in the big books on the kidney that are described in the preface and in a number of physiology texts such as the following:

R. F. Pitts. *Physiology of the kidney and body fluids,* 3rd ed. Chicago: Year Book Medical Publishers, 1974.

H. Valtin. *Renal function: Mechanisms preserving fluid and solute balance in health.* Boston: Little, Brown, 1973.

4
Sodium and Water Homeostasis in the Body

Many people think of the kidneys only as organs that dispose of bodily wastes. While this is an important function, it is only one part of a much broader responsibility the kidneys have—that of maintaining internal homeostasis in the body. As part of this responsibility the kidneys must regulate the excretion of many substances not ordinarily thought of as wastes, such as sodium and water.

PRESERVING THE INTERNAL ENVIRONMENT

Living cells are quite fussy about the environment in which they live. The conditions have to be just right and must not vary greatly or the cells will fail to function or may even die. Microorganisms, for instance, grow more readily at some temperatures than others. At low temperatures they stop growing and may die, and high temperatures will destroy them. In a similar way living cells are dependent on the chemical conditions (the concentrations of many different substances) in their surroundings and they get sick or die if there is much change from ideal conditions.

Most biological historians believe life on Earth originated in the sea. Because of its immense size and the properties of water, the sea provided these one-celled organisms with stable conditions that could be found nowhere else. The sun could shine or storms could blow, but the chemical environment in the sea would be as little affected as a supertanker that has been rammed by a canoe.

When some animals moved onto the land many years later, they left the protective stability of the sea to face a cruel and fickle environment where it might be too hot or too cold, too dry or too wet, and where vital chemicals such as sodium chloride might be in short supply. How could their cells survive in such a place? It appears that the multicellular organisms made this possible by surrounding their cells with an internal sea where conditions could be kept stable despite fluctuations in the weather outside. This notion, generally accepted now, was popularized by the French physiologist Claude Bernard. The constant *milieu intérieur* (internal environment) that he described corresponds pretty much to what modern physiologists call the extracellular fluid.

The cells of modern higher animals are probably even more fastidious about their immediate environment than were the cells of simpler organisms. They are specialized for complex functions such as nerve conduction, muscle contraction, and metabolism, and they cannot be bothered, nor are they equipped, to protect themselves against environmental changes. Rather, they are able to carry out their complicated tasks only because an ideal and stable internal environment is provided for them by other cells in the system. It is the role of the kidneys, themselves specialists, to maintain constant and optimal conditions in the extracellular fluid with respect to fluid volume, osmolality and pH, plus many electrolytes and waste products. In this chapter we shall be concerned with the maintenance of optimal volume and osmolality in the extracellular fluid.

WHY ARE VOLUME AND OSMOLALITY IMPORTANT?

First, let's look at the volume of the extracellular fluid. The extracellular fluid includes the plasma water in which blood cells are suspended, and its volume is critical for efficient performance of the circulatory system. If there is not enough extracellular fluid, there may be too little blood volume to fill capillaries and perfuse all the tissues adequately; if the deficiency becomes dire enough, it may result in one of the situations referred to as *shock*. Too much extracellular fluid can also cause problems; the extra fluid is likely to enter the interstitial spaces between capillaries and body cells, causing swelling of the tissues (edema) and increasing the distance necessary for diffusion of nutrients and waste products between capillaries and cells. These problems are illustrated diagrammatically in Figure 4-1. Too much extracellular fluid may also overload the circulatory system, causing cardiac decompensation and accumulation of edema in the lungs, where it may interfere with gas transport.

The maintenance of optimal osmolality in the extracellular fluid is equally important, because the cells, for the most part, have no way to regulate their own osmolality. There have been a few experiments suggesting that certain cells, under special conditions, are capable of some osmotic regulation—but it is reasonable to believe that the vast majority of cells under virtually all conditions have no osmotic regulating ability. Their membranes are freely permeable to water, which enters and leaves the cells in response to osmotic forces, so that effective osmolality remains the same inside and outside the cells. So if a cell is placed in an environment of high osmolality, water will

HYPOVOLEMIA   NORMOVOLEMIA   HYPERVOLEMIA

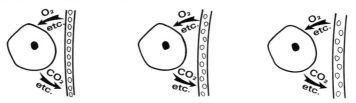

Figure 4-1. The effect of extracellular fluid volume on capillary fullness and the fluid space between cells and their capillaries.

leave the cell, and the cell will shrink until its osmolality rises to equal that of the environment. Under conditions of low surrounding osmolality, on the other hand, cells will take up water and swell. These changes are illustrated in Figure 4-2. It is obvious that the volume of cells as well as their osmolality is determined by the effective osmolality of the extracellular fluid. Some cells are especially vulnerable to damage from abnormal shrinking and swelling. The brain, for instance, is enclosed in the rigid skull and has no place to go if its cells try to expand in response to a decrease in environmental osmolality. Instead, the pressure rises within the skull, often with disastrous consequences.

Before we examine how the kidneys maintain normal osmotic conditions in the extracellular fluid, we must come to grips with . . .

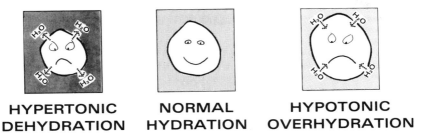

HYPERTONIC   NORMAL   HYPOTONIC
DEHYDRATION   HYDRATION   OVERHYDRATION

Figure 4-2. The effect on cells of changes in the osmolality of the fluid around them. The cell on the left is in an environment of abnormally high osmolality, while the cell on the right is being subjected to an environment of low osmolality.

THE CRITICAL ROLE OF SODIUM

Sodium and the anions that accompany it occupy a pivotal position in osmotic and volume regulation in the extracellular fluid. There are two major reasons for this:

1. There is so much of it. Under normal circumstances sodium and its anions make up over 90% of the osmotic particles in the extracellular fluid.
2. Sodium is actively excluded from cells (just as potassium is actively sequestered within cells).

So the osmotic effect that sodium in the extracellular fluid has upon cells is in direct proportion to the concentration of the sodium, since there is virtually no sodium within the cells to balance the effect of the sodium outside. This behavior of sodium is in contrast to that of solutes that diffuse into cells, such as urea. Since the concentration of urea inside cells can come into equilibrium with the concentration outside, urea does not exert an osmotic effect on cells (under equilibrium conditions, at least) and is therefore not an effective osmotic particle, even though it may raise the measured osmolality of the extracellular fluid.

Because there is so much sodium compared with other solutes, and because sodium remains outside cells, the osmolality that affects cellular hydration (the effective osmolality of the extracellular fluid) is almost entirely due to the concentration of sodium and its anions. Therefore one can assume with considerable confidence that a low concentration of sodium in the extracellular fluid (measured in the blood serum)* means that the fluid is hypo-osmotic. Similarly a high concentration of sodium means that the extracellular fluid is hypertonic, meaning that body cells are also hypertonic and somewhat shrunken from loss of water. Where an osmometer is not available to measure the osmolality of the plasma water, a reasonable approximation of effective osmolality can usually be made by multiplying the plasma sodium concentration by 2.

The general rule that the plasma sodium concentration is an accurate reflection of plasma and extracellular fluid osmolality has exceptions worth remembering. The most common of these occurs when there is a gross elevation of plasma glucose levels, as in poorly controlled diabetes mellitus. Due to the basic metabolic abnormality of diabetes mellitus, glucose cannot enter cells readily; so, being largely confined to the extracellular fluid, it exerts an effective osmotic influence on cells. (Plasma osmolality rises by 10 mOsm/kg of water when the plasma glucose rises by 180 mg/dl.) As the extracellular fluid becomes hyperosmotic because of high glucose levels, water flows from the cells into the extracellular fluid to maintain osmotic equilibrium. This flow of water from the cells dilutes the sodium concentration in the extracellular fluid, often to subnormal levels—yet the total osmolality in the extracellular fluid is increased when both sodium and glucose are taken into account. And the cells, of course, are shrunken and dehydrated.

---

*The concentration of sodium in the extracellular fluid is not really identical to that in serum because of the Donnan effect, explained in Chapter 1, but the difference is not of consequence for our purposes and will be ignored here. Serum and plasma sodium concentrations are essentially identical, and we shall use them interchangeably, though the actual determination is customarily performed on serum.

Plasma sodium may also be a misleading guide to effective osmolality in the rare instances when there are grossly abnormal levels of either protein or lipids in the plasma. Sodium is dissolved in the plasma water, which normally accounts for about 93% of the plasma volume (the rest being mostly dissolved protein). Extremely high levels of protein or lipoprotein can reduce this percentage of plasma that is water. Even though the concentration of sodium in the plasma water is normal, there is less plasma water and therefore less sodium per 100 ml of plasma under these circumstances, and the laboratory will report a reduced number of milliequivalents (or millimoles) of sodium per liter of serum. The osmotic effect on the cells is normal, however, so long as the sodium concentration in the plasma *water* is normal.

Although it is well to have these exceptions filed away in one's memory, it is far more important to remember the general principle that plasma sodium concentration determines osmolality under most circumstances. And it follows that the responsibility of the kidneys to regulate the osmolality of the extracellular fluid is, in effect, a responsibility to regulate the concentration of sodium. This is accomplished in a way that is different from what you might expect.

TENDING THE TANK

The kidneys may be compared, then, to an engineer who is in charge of a very important tank of solution—the extracellular fluid (Fig. 4-3). He does not have complete control of the tank. Several times each day the gastrointestinal gremlin comes around and pours unpredictable amounts of sodium salts or water or both into it. Some water is lost from the tank by evaporation, and at times some sodium and water may be lost by other routes, but our engineer controls the major route for removal of sodium and water from the tank. His job is to keep the volume and sodium concentration constant in the tank, if possible, in spite of what is done to upset them.

If we had to design a system to control the volume and the sodium concentration in the tank, most of us would probably arrange things so that water would be removed when the volume in the tank becomes too great, and sodium would be removed when its concentration becomes too high. That's a nice, logical idea—but *forget it!* The system doesn't work that way, although many medical students and doctors apparently think that it does.

On the contrary, a massive amount of experimental evidence indicates that renal sodium excretion is controlled by changes in the *volume* of the extracellular fluid—not by its sodium concentration. And the renal excretion of water appears to be governed primarily by the *osmolality* (read sodium concentration) of the extracellular fluid—not by its volume. These basic relationships, summarized in Figure 4-4, account for the responses of normal subjects to the illustrative situations that follow.

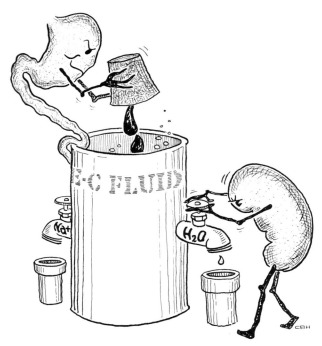

Figure 4-3. The kidney as chief engineer and protector of a threatened internal environment.

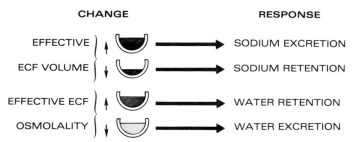

Figure 4-4. The basic influences regulating the excretion of sodium and water by the kidneys. (But see also Fig. 4-5 for an important refinement.)

Situation

Decreased volume of extracellular fluid
Elevated serum sodium concentration

Renal Response

Sodium retention (little sodium in urine)
Water retention (concentrated urine)
Note that the elevation of serum sodium does not cause sodium excretion.

Situation

Increased volume of extracellular fluid
Decreased serum sodium concentration

Renal Response

Sodium excretion (much sodium in urine)
Water excretion (dilute urine)
The decreased serum sodium concentration does not prevent the sodium excretion that occurs in response to volume expansion.

Situation

Increased volume of extracellular fluid
Elevated serum sodium concentration

Renal Response

Sodium excretion (much sodium in urine)
Some water retention (concentrated urine)
Note that the increased volume of extracellular fluid does not cause the kidneys to pour out water freely; they are responding to the elevated serum osmolality. But for reasons to be explained shortly, the urine will be less concentrated here than in the first situation, where the volume of the extracellular fluid was decreased.

In the examples we have just considered, you may have been disturbed by the fact that the amount of sodium in the urine and the concentration of the urine do not always go in the same direction, an apparent contradiction. Though sodium concentration is closely linked to osmolality in the extracellular fluid, urine contains other solutes, primarily urea, that may contribute more osmotic particles than sodium and its anions. Thus a urine of high osmolality may be produced that contains virtually no sodium. Conversely, a dilute urine may have a low sodium concentration but contain a large total amount of sodium if the volume of the urine is great.

The control arrangements described here may at first appear illogical, but with a little reflection you'll be able to see that the system works fine this way and tends to bring the extracellular fluid back toward normal following various disturbances. The kidneys are aided in this task by the fact that an increase in the effective osmolality of the extracellular fluid typically produces the sensation of thirst, which leads to increased water intake if water is available.

Let's see how this system maintains internal homeostasis in the face of various types of attack. Suppose, for instance, that a college student consumes a large box of pretzels all by himself. This substantial intake of sodium chloride causes compartmental changes (described in Chapter 1 and Figs. 1-2 and 1-3) and sets in motion a number of responses. Though many of these events actually take place simultaneously, it is easier to think of them as a sequence:

1. Following absorption from the gastrointestinal tract, the sodium and chloride are confined to the extracellular fluid space, since they are excluded from cells. Their addition raises the osmolality of the extracellular fluid.

2. In response to the higher osmolality of the extracellular fluid, water diffuses from the cells until osmotic equilibrium is reached between intracellular and extracellular fluid. Thus the extracellular fluid compartment enlarges while the intracellular compartment shrinks. If total body water has not been increased, this transfer of water leaves both compartments somewhat hyperosmotic.

3. Since hyperosmolality stimulates thirst, the student drinks water (or beer) until internal osmolality is reduced to normal. The ingested water distributes itself osmotically between extracellular fluid and cell water. When normal osmolality is restored, the intracellular fluid will be back to its original volume, but the extracellular fluid will be expanded because of the extra sodium and chloride it contains.

4. The expansion of the extracellular fluid stimulates renal excretion of sodium, which must take an anion, usually chloride, with it.

5. If sodium is excreted in excess relative to water, the osmolality of the extracellular fluid starts to fall. This stimulates the excretion of water so that normal osmolality is maintained.

6. The sequence ends when normal volume and osmolality are restored in the extracellular fluid. At this point the kidneys have eliminated the sodium chloride ingested originally, plus the water that was taken subsequently.

In a healthy person all these events will have taken place with only minor changes in the volume and sodium concentration of the extracellular fluid.

Suppose on the other hand that our student, instead of eating pretzels, drinks a large quantity of water. This will distribute itself osmotically to both intracellular and extracellular compartments, though more to the larger intracellular compartment, reducing the osmolality of both. In response to the decreased osmolality, the kidneys will be stimulated to excrete water, and a dilute urine will be produced until the extra water is eliminated. Since there was some expansion of the extracellular fluid following water ingestion, there might be some stimulus also to excrete sodium—which might not be appropriate under these circumstances. But typically osmotic regulation is so sensitive and excretion of water so efficient that the extra water can be eliminated before very much expansion of the extracellular fluid has taken place, especially since the intracellular compartment gets the lion's share of an ingested water load.

We have seen how the system responds to an excess of sodium or water.

The same general control principles can be seen at work in situations where sodium or water are deficient. An abnormal loss of sodium is usually accompanied—up to a point—by a corresponding loss of water, maintaining normal osmolality. The resulting shrinkage of the extracellular fluid stimulates normal kidneys to reabsorb sodium avidly, yielding almost none to the urine. Similarly a deficiency of water alone raises serum osmolality, stimulating the kidneys to produce a hypertonic urine, thus minimizing the further loss of water. Under these circumstances of deficient sodium or water, the kidneys cannot restore conditions to normal, since they cannot replace what has been lost, but they can minimize the amount of damage that is done to internal homeostasis.

BUT IN THE REAL WORLD . . .

It seems a shame to mess up this nice, tidy control system by adding new factors, but unfortunately things are a bit more complicated than we have described them. Here's the problem: Although the effective osmolality of the extracellular fluid appears to determine how much water the kidneys excrete or retain in the body under most circumstances, there is convincing evidence that abnormalities in the *volume* of the extracellular fluid may also influence renal water excretion. For instance, an otherwise normal subject with low serum sodium concentration should produce a dilute urine to rid the body of excess water and restore normal osmolality. But if this subject also has a significant reduction in the *volume* of the extracellular fluid, water excretion is likely to be inhibited; the urine will be less dilute than we would expect from osmotic considerations alone, or it may even be concentrated.

Why is this happening? From an adaptive point of view it may make sense. We are considering a subject who has too little extracellular fluid with a higher-than-normal ratio of water to sodium, that is, a low serum sodium concentration. Excretion of water to raise the sodium concentration would mean some loss of water from the already depleted extracellular fluid (though most would come from within the cells), reducing its volume even further. Perhaps the failure to excrete more water under these circumstances means that the physiological mechanisms have decided that the body needs all of its remaining extracellular fluid more than it needs restoration of normal osmolality. Whatever the "motives," the influence of volume depletion on renal water excretion is a well-established and clinically important phenomenon.

Conversely, there is evidence that volume expansion of the extracellular fluid facilitates the excretion of water, though this effect is less impressive than that of a reduced volume.

So it looks as though some extra arrows will have to be added to Figure 4-4 to reflect the influence of extracellular fluid volume on water excretion. The amended version is shown as Figure 4-5.

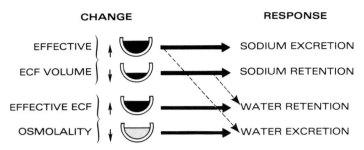

Figure 4-5. The basic influences regulating the excretion of sodium and water by the kidneys, including the influence of extracellular fluid volume on water excretion.

HOW DO THE KIDNEYS KNOW WHAT TO DO?

We have seen how the renal excretion of sodium and water is governed by the volume and osmotic state of the extracellular fluid. But how are these factors monitored, and how do the kidneys find out about them? In situations like this it makes physiologists happy if they can find a specific, localized receptor that senses the variable to be regulated. The search for an osmolality-receptor has been gratifying, but efforts to identify *the* volume-receptor have been quite frustrating.

The Osmoreceptor

More than 30 years ago Verney injected concentrated saline solutions into the carotid arteries of dogs and observed that this caused a prompt increase in the urine osmolality. The same solutions injected into peripheral veins had much less effect on urine osmolality. Verney concluded—quite correctly, as it turned out—that there is a receptor in the vascular bed of the carotid artery that senses elevations of osmolality in the plasma and causes the release of a hormone that tells the kidneys to conserve water. The *antidiuretic hormone* was subsequently identified and synthesized by du Vigneaud and co-workers. It appears to be produced in the hypothalamus by the cells of the supraoptic and possibly the paraventricular nuclei. Perhaps as part of a larger carrier molecule it travels down the axons of these cells to the posterior pituitary (neurohypophysis), where it is stored until needed. Its release into the circulation for passage to the kidneys is evidently triggered by the osmoreceptor (which may reside in the same cells that produce the hormone) and sometimes by other influences.

Antidiuretic hormone, or simply ADH, is also known as *vasopressin* because it is a potent vasoconstrictor when used in higher concentrations than those usually present in the blood. It is a small peptide molecule, consisting of eight or nine amino acids, depending on how you count cystine/cysteine (Fig. 4-6). Although it is frustrating to students to have multiple words for the same

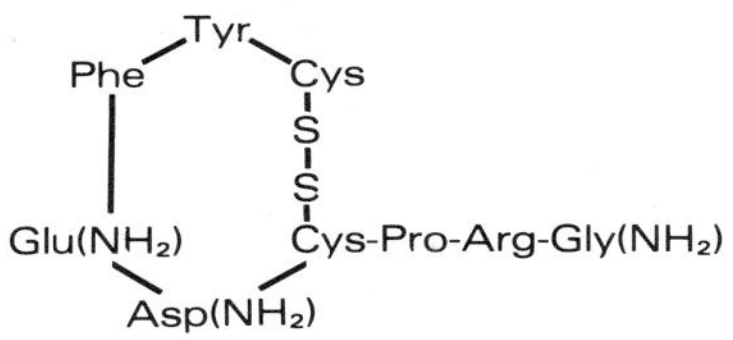

Figure 4-6. Amino-acid sequence in arginine vasopressin, the antidiuretic hormone of humans and most other mammals.

hormone, both ADH and vasopressin are used so commonly that you had better learn both names.

Concentration and dilution of the urine may be affected significantly by factors other than vasopressin, but under normal circumstances this hormone appears to be the dominant influence in determining the osmolality of the urine. Its mechanism of action in the kidneys will be discussed in Chapter 6.

Where Are You, Volume-Receptor?

In contrast to the osmoreceptor, the volume-receptor has eluded discovery despite numerous laboratory experiments designed to locate it. Investigators have removed various organs such as the liver from experimental animals and have denervated suspected receptor areas, but the animals are still able to respond appropriately to changes in the volume of the extracellular fluid. Are we any wiser than we were before? Well, perhaps a little. By a process of exclusion, some reasonable hypotheses have emerged from these experiments.

One such hypothesis is that the volume-receptor is diffuse and includes much of the vascular system. According to this view, receptors in the walls of the blood vessels sense the fullness and stretch of the vessels and convey this information to the central nervous system, from which it is transmitted to the kidneys over efferent nerves or conceivably by means of hormones. Any such stretch receptors in the high-pressure arterial system would obviously not be measuring the volume of extracellular fluid directly; rather, they would be sensing the blood volume, which is related, and also the ability of the heart to keep the arterial vessels filled and under appropriate pressure.

It has also been suggested that the kidneys themselves are volume-receptors. This would explain the failure of many previous experiments to identify the volume-receptor. The kidneys could not be removed in those experiments because they were needed; their excretion or nonexcretion of sodium told the investigator how the extracellular volume was being sensed. It seems quite possible that a receptor role could reside in the specialized arteriolar cells of the juxtaglomerular apparatus; these cells might be influenced by the fullness of the arterial system to produce or release more or less renin, depending on the circumstances. And renin, we know, is a hormone that initiates a series of reactions leading to production of the sodium-retaining hormone aldosterone. But the kidneys are unlikely to be the *only* volume-receptor because experimental reduction of the blood pressure in the renal arteries does not always prevent the excretion of large amounts of sodium in response to expansion of the extracellular fluid. In this situation it appears that the kidneys must be getting messages from somewhere else about the state of the extracellular fluid volume.

Most of the hypotheses mentioned so far suggest that the volume-receptor is really sensing the fullness of some part of the circulatory system. There is indeed good reason to believe that the perception of volume is influenced by circulatory factors, as will be discussed next, but it may be more complicated than that. For instance, intravenous infusion of saline solution into an experimental animal results in more excretion of sodium than does an infusion of albumin that produces the same increase in the plasma volume. If the volume-receptor were concerned only with *circulatory* fullness, both infusions should be followed by the same amount of renal sodium excretion.

Obviously our quest for a simple, localized volume-receptor has led us into a morass; no one explanation seems to account for all the evidence available. It may just be that many different messages from different parts of the body contribute to the physiological perception of extracellular fluid volume.

FALSE SIGNALS AND SWOLLEN ANKLES

Under normal circumstances extra sodium chloride given to an individual will not produce a large or long-term expansion of extracellular fluid volume, since it will be excreted promptly as already described. Yet circumstances are commonly encountered in which people with kidneys that appear normal may have gross expansion of the extracellular fluid volume, usually manifested by edema, swelling of the tissues. How does this happen? Typically, in such situations the kidneys will be found to be excreting relatively little sodium; they do not seem to be responding appropriately to the obvious enlargement of the extracellular fluid volume. Given the presence of edema, this is not so surprising. After all, if the kidneys had been responding to the enlarging extracellular fluid volume by increasing the excretion of sodium, the edema would not have developed.

What has gone wrong with the finely tuned mechanisms for keeping the volume of the extracellular fluid just right? In many edema-forming situations the kidneys appear to be perfectly normal—except that they behave *as though* the extracellular fluid were depleted, rather than expanded. This has led physiologists to the conclusion that the kidneys are responding to false signals; that is, the volume-receptors are telling the kidneys that the extracellular fluid volume is low, even though it is actually enlarged. It is easy to see how this could happen. After all, the possible volume-receptors we discussed would not really measure volume, but rather pressure or stretch (fullness) in some part of the vascular bed. And edema often occurs in situations where there may be decreased fullness in the vascular system.

Rather than abandon the whole concept that sodium excretion responds to expansion of the extracellular fluid volume—which works well most of the time—physiologists have found some weasel-words to cover these situations where volume is perceived by the receptors as decreased even though it is actually expanded. In such situations it is said that the *effective* extracellular fluid volume or *effective* plasma volume is decreased. Presumably this effective volume is the fullness or stretch of the vascular system that the volume-receptors are actually monitoring.

EXAMPLES OF EDEMA

First, a few comments about edema in general. As used here, edema means the accumulation of interstitial fluid in body tissues sufficient to be detected by physical examination. Edema is usually noted first in the ankles and/or legs at the end of the day because gravitational forces in dependent parts of the body increase the tendency there for plasma water to leave the capillaries. At times edema may be due primarily to local factors, in which case there may be only a small increase in total extracellular fluid. But edema is often a reflection of a generalized increase in extracellular fluid volume. Careful measurements in such situations have shown that several liters or more of extra fluid may accumulate in a normal adult before edema becomes noticeable.

Renal retention of sodium plays a critical role in the development of edema (except perhaps where edema is very small in amount and due entirely to local factors). A corresponding amount of water is retained with the sodium so that edematous patients usually have a normal plasma sodium concentration. Occasionally water excretion is also impaired significantly, presumably in response to a perception of decreased effective volume, and hyponatremia may develop. Even in the presence of a decreased plasma sodium concentration, however, it has been shown that patients with edema have an increase in the total amount of sodium in the body.

Cardiac Edema

Edema is common in individuals with cardiac insufficiency. It seems reasonable to suppose that decreased cardiac output results in decreased fullness in the arterial system and that this is interpreted by volume-receptors as diminished blood volume; in short, the effective blood volume is decreased. The kidneys are then programmed to reabsorb sodium very efficiently, just as they would be if there had been a real loss of extracellular fluid. The retained sodium (and water retained with it) does expand the plasma volume, but it also makes its way into the interstitial space, forming edema. This tendency to form edema is promoted also by the elevation in venous and capillary pressure often found in the presence of a failing heart. Despite an actual increase in the volume of the extracellular fluid and plasma water, the effective volume remains low because the failing heart cannot pump well enough to restore normal fullness or stretch to the arterial bed. The retained fluid usually makes things worse, in fact, causing pulmonary edema, impaired peripheral capillary exchange, and sometimes reduced cardiac output as a result of diastolic overfilling.

Here is a situation in which some normal physiological mechanisms, designed to protect against depletion of extracellular fluid and plasma volume, appear to be counteradaptive in the presence of heart failure. Patients with cardiac edema usually benefit from judicious use of diuretic drugs to block renal retention of sodium.

Nephrotic Edema

Certain renal diseases are characterized by the loss of large quantities of serum proteins, especially albumin, into the urine, although the kidneys may be functionally intact otherwise. Patients with these *nephrotic* diseases typically demonstrate renal sodium retention and edema.

The generally accepted explanation for this edema formation is as follows: The loss of large amounts of albumin into the urine may exceed the synthetic capacity of the liver and result in a decrease of serum albumin concentration. And this decreases the oncotic pressure of plasma, resulting in a loss of plasma water to the interstitial space. The actual volume of plasma is thus reduced, triggering the volume-receptors, which direct the kidneys to retain sodium. Continued dietary intake of sodium in the face of greatly diminished renal excretion causes formation of additional extracellular fluid. Some of this may remain in the plasma, since there continues to be an equilibrium between plasma and interstitial fluid, even though the proportions are changed in the presence of a low serum albumin concentration. But most of the newly formed extracellular fluid will be lost to the interstitial space because of the low plasma oncotic pressure which allowed plasma water to escape in the first place. So the cycle continues: More sodium is retained and more extracellular fluid formed, but it does not restore the plasma volume, so the stimulus for sodium retention continues, and the edema caused by increased interstitial fluid may grow to massive proportions.

In this situation normal volume-protecting mechanisms are frustrated because most of the retained sodium and water will not stay in the plasma compartment where they are needed. Yet, if even a little of the retained fluid remains in the plasma, the adaptation is not entirely futile. Herein lies the dilemma of treating patients with nephrotic edema. They do not like the edema, which is disfiguring, uncomfortable and sometimes even disabling. The physician may be able to get rid of the edema with diuretic drugs, but in order to eliminate the unwanted interstitial fluid he risks some further reduction of the already reduced plasma volume, with the possible consequences of hypotension or inadequate perfusion of vital organs or both.

Should he risk it? There is no easy answer. The choice will be influenced by how much discomfort the patient is having from his edema and, if treatment is undertaken, how he responds to it. Many nephrotic patients will tolerate the gradual removal of large amounts of edema with no apparent circulatory deterioration. But the physician undertaking such treatment must be aware that he is using diuretic drugs to circumvent a physiological mechanism that may be protecting the patient from something worse than edema. Caution and continuing observation during treatment are mandatory.

Recently an alternative explanation for the formation of nephrotic edema has been proposed. It has been suggested that nephrotic patients retain sodium because their intrarenal mechanisms for sodium excretion are disturbed by the same disease processes that cause the urinary loss of albumin, or perhaps because albumin in the tubular fluid interferes with sodium excretion. This explanation would make renal retention of sodium a primary event in edema formation rather than a secondary response to the loss of plasma water into interstitial tissue. Plasma volume would be expanded—not contracted—and the proponents of this view point out that some nephrotic patients do appear to have normal or increased plasma volumes. If this proves to be the case generally, treatment of such patients with diuretics will become physiologically respectable.

Fluid Retention in Cirrhosis of the Liver

It is fairly common for patients with cirrhosis of the liver to develop ascites, a collection of free fluid within the peritoneal cavity. This fluid resembles extracellular fluid in its electrolyte composition. Some of these patients also have edema in the extremities and elsewhere.

The traditional explanation for these findings has related the ascites to increased venous pressure in the portal circulation caused by obstruction to portal outflow within the diseased liver. According to this interpretation, extracellular fluid escapes from the small vessels of the portal circulation—especially those in the liver capsule—into the peritoneal cavity at an accelerated rate because of increased capillary hydrostatic pressure. Low serum albumin concentration caused by decreased hepatic synthesis of albumin may promote this loss of fluid. When fluid enters the peritoneal cavity at a rate that exceeds the rate at which the lymphatic system can return it to the circulation, ascites forms. This process tends to reduce plasma volume, and the same mechanisms described for nephrotic edema (the generally accepted explanation for nephrotic edema) then operate to promote renal sodium retention and restore plasma volume. But a significant part of the retained sodium and water may escape into the ascites, and so the process continues, often with formation of many liters of ascites. In short, this view regards renal sodium retention as compensatory, a result of ascites formation. When these patients also have edema, it could be the result of decreased serum albumin concentrations and possibly elevated pressure in the inferior vena cava.

However, some recent evidence indicates that the disease process in the liver may have a direct effect on renal tubules through mechanisms unknown, stimulating them to reabsorb sodium without any decrease in the plasma volume. Thus there would be an initial *increase* in the plasma volume. With continued sodium and water accumulation, the retained fluid would seek to leave the vascular system, and the part of the vascular system most vulnerable to such escape would be the portal bed, where venous pressure is increased. So ascites formation, according to this point of view, would be secondary to a primary process of renal sodium retention. Proponents of this view point to evidence that measured plasma volume is often increased—not decreased—in patients with cirrhosis of the liver.

The jury of expert opinion is still out on this controversy. Meanwhile it is difficult to decide whether the renal sodium retention so characteristic of patients with cirrhosis and ascites is an attempt to protect the plasma volume against dangerous depletion or whether it is causing the whole fluid problem. One thing seems fairly certain from extensive clinical experience: Anyone who attempts to remove the accumulated fluid from these patients in a hurry is courting disaster, for such efforts are often attended by rapid deterioration in renal and hepatic function. If fluid is to be removed at all, it must be done very slowly.

The three examples of fluid retention just mentioned, cardiac failure, nephrotic syndrome, and cirrhosis of the liver, illustrate how massive amounts of extracellular fluid may accumulate, given the appropriate physiological signals, despite the presence of good kidney function. Two other types of edema should be mentioned, though they are not in the same category.

Edema Due to Local Factors

Edema may form locally in response to inflammation or to obstruction of venous or lymphatic outflow. For example, it may be found in a leg following deep vein thrombosis or in an arm following surgery that interrupts drainage channels in the axilla. The mechanism is presumably a disturbance of Starling's capillary forces as a result of elevated local venous pressure. The balance of sodium and water in the rest of the body is not disturbed, though the kidneys will retain enough extra sodium and water to make up for what has been lost from the vascular system in the area of edema.

Local edema is most logically treated by measures to improve local venous and lymphatic drainage. Diuretics are sometimes used and may help a little, though this approach is basically unphysiological; after all, it means inducing some depletion of the extracellular fluid volume in all the rest of the body in order to promote the resorption of edema fluid from just one area.

Edema with Renal Failure

Edema due to retention of sodium is often found in patients with renal failure. In this setting we do not have to look for tricky false signals and physiological protective mechanisms to explain what is happening. In fact, the physiological mechanisms in chronic renal failure are probably responding appropriately to the increased extracellular fluid volume and telling the kidneys to excrete as much sodium as possible. And the kidneys—what is left of them—appear to be responding. The problem is that there is simply not enough functioning kidney tissue left to do the job. So even though each remaining nephron excretes (i.e., fails to reabsorb) much more sodium than it ever would under normal circumstances, the total excretion of sodium may still be less than the dietary intake of sodium.

The resulting fluid accumulation is distinctly unphysiological and can cause the patient major problems, such as hypertension and pulmonary edema as well as swelling of legs and other tissues. Methods for treating this problem will be discussed in the chapter on chronic renal failure.

By this time it must be apparent that edema and ascites are symptoms of varied disturbances whose common feature happens to be the retention of abnormal amounts of sodium and water. The underlying problems are quite different, as are the mechanisms of sodium retention. Especially important is the fact that in some cases the fluid retention may have a real compensatory role in supporting the volume of a depleted compartment, while in other cases it is futile or actually makes matters worse. It follows, of course, that removing the extra fluid by the use of diuretics may be harmful to some patients and very helpful to others. So it is important to consider the underlying problem and mechanisms in each case in order to predict what will happen if the extra fluid is removed. *Diuretics should not be given blindly to everyone with swollen legs.*

INTAKE OF SODIUM AND WATER—THE OTHER SIDE OF THE EQUATION

Very little has been said thus far about *intake* of sodium and water. Yet it should be apparent that the maintenance of ideal quantities of sodium and water in the body depends on what comes in as well as what goes out. Since some losses from the system are inevitable, especially in the case of water, there should be a mechanism to ensure that at least enough comes in to offset obligatory losses. Ideally there should also be mechanisms to turn off the intake of sodium and water if they threaten to unbalance the system.

But only one of these mechanisms, the thirst mechanism that protects against water depletion, seems to play an important and consistent role in all mammals. One reason is that eating and drinking are not controlled exclusively by physiological needs. Especially in humans, these forms of behavior are influenced by personal and cultural taste preferences as well as by economic, social, and psychological factors. Another reason may be that under normal conditions the kidneys can excrete sodium and water so efficiently that close control of intake is unnecessary, since precise regulation can be accomplished at the excretory level. This arrangement works beautifully most of the time, but it can cause real trouble if the excretory mechanisms fail.

Water Intake—The Thirst Mechanism

Everyone is familiar with the sensation of thirst. Under appropriate circumstances it protects animals from dehydration by creating an extremely potent drive to ingest water. The stimuli causing thirst appear to be much the same as those that promote the release of vasopressin and thus the conservation of water by the kidneys. The most demonstrable of these stimuli is an increase in effective osmolality of the extracellular fluid. The osmolality is sensed by an osmoreceptor in the hypothalamic portion of the brain, perhaps close to or identical with the osmoreceptor that regulates vasopressin. From the osmoreceptor, messages travel over neuronal pathways, probably via an integrating center, to the level of consciousness where they are interpreted as thirst.

Like the release of vasopressin, thirst may also appear in response to depletion of the effective extracellular fluid or plasma volume. Some investigators believe that the renin-angiotensin system is involved in transmitting this message, while others have produced evidence that beta-adrenergic stimuli play a role. Whatever the mechanisms, volume stimuli appear to be less consistent and reliable than osmotic stimuli in producing the sensation of thirst. This is quite apparent in humans; for example, some persons who have suffered a significant loss of blood complain of thirst, while others do not.

Since thirst and the release of vasopressin are both stimulated by the same conditions, it has been suggested that vasopressin may cause the perception of thirst. It's a reasonable idea, but apparently not true. Humans and animals who lack this hormone are found occasionally, but they are able to get mighty thirsty without it.

So much for the mechanisms that stimulate water intake by turning on the sensation of thirst. It should also be possible to turn off thirst when water is not needed, and the well-hydrated human or animal usually does indeed show a lack of interest in water. But circumstances are found in which humans who lack the known stimuli for thirst—whose extracellular fluid may in fact be expanded and hypo-osmotic—continue to drink water, often to their considerable detriment. In some situations, such as cardiac insufficiency, it may be argued that such people are responding to false signals set up by a decrease in their effective plasma volume—just as their kidneys respond to reduced effective volume by retaining sodium and sometimes water.

But what of the patient on chronic dialysis with nonfunctioning kidneys who insists that he is thirsty and continues to drink water and other liquids even though his serum sodium concentration is low and his effective plasma volume appears by all indications to be enlarged? Such behavior, which is rather common, is hard to explain in physiological terms alone. Perhaps we must conclude that in such cases the psychological or habitual drives for fluid ingestion have overcome any physiological defenses against excessive water intake. And it appears that these physiological defenses may be almost nonexistent. Since the kidneys under normal circumstances can excrete enormous amounts of unwanted water, frugal Mother Nature evidently did not consider it necessary to provide a strong defense mechanism against excessive water intake.

In summary, the thirst mechanism regulates water intake by responding strongly to hyperosmotic stimuli and less consistently to volume-deficiency stimuli. But thirst may be present even in the absence of these stimuli, suggesting that nonphysiological influences may also be important.

The Dubious Regulation of Sodium Intake

Sodium is so important to the internal environment that we would not expect its acquisition to be left to chance. Indeed, there is good evidence that some animals have an appetite for salt which is directly related to needs. For example, sodium-depleted rats or sheep take more sodium when it is available than do non-sodium-depleted controls, and the amount of additional sodium they take is in proportion to their deficit. However, humans in general are not as smart as rats and sheep when it comes to recognizing their need for sodium. Under circumstances of sodium depletion some humans experience a craving for salt, but many others do not. They may have major symptoms of sodium depletion, such as lethargy, muscle cramps, and general loss of taste, but the strong desire for salt that would be physiologically appropriate under the circumstances is just not there.

However, many animals, including humans, have a taste preference for salt whether they need it at the moment or not, and most human diets contain a surfeit of sodium. So an intake in excess of actual needs is usually assured. The kidneys do the real regulating by conserving sodium avidly when necessary or—as is more often the case—by discarding excess sodium in the urine.

But what happens when the renal capacity to excrete sodium is impaired or destroyed? Apparently the taste preference for sodium goes right on (at least in humans) and causes an accumulation of extracellular fluid that can be of disastrous proportions. As was the case with water intake, we appear to lack a mechanism to turn off sodium intake when we do not need it and cannot handle it.

In short, adequate sodium intake is generally assured by a natural taste preference, and this appetite for salt is intensified in some animals under conditions of sodium depletion. In humans, at least, there appears to be no inhibition of sodium intake even when it is already present in excess.

BIBLIOGRAPHY

J. T. Fitzsimons. The physiological basis of thirst. *Kidney Int.* 10: 3–11, 1976.
The entire issue of Kidney International *for July 1976 (Vol. 10, No. 1), is devoted to a symposium on water metabolism.*

M. Levy. The pathophysiology of sodium balance. *Hosp. Prac.* 13: 95–106, November 1978.

G. L. Robertson, R. L. Shelton, and S. Athar. The osmoregulation of vasopressin. *Kidney Int.* 10: 25–37, 1976.

R. W. Schrier and T. Berl. Nonosmolar factors affecting renal water excretion. *N. Engl. J. Med.* 292: 81–88, 1975.

5
How the Kidneys Regulate Sodium Excretion

In the preceding chapter we saw that the renal excretion of sodium appears to be governed by the actual or at least the effective volume of the extracellular fluid or circulation or both. An increase in these volumes leads to increased renal sodium excretion, while shrinkage of the extracellular fluid or circulatory volume results in renal sodium retention. In this chapter we shall deal with some of the mechanisms within the kidneys by which these adjustments in sodium excretion are made.

The precise regulation of sodium excretion to match the needs of the body is an awesome and challenging responsibility. Consider what is required: The human diet may contain anywhere from virtually no sodium to several hundred milliequivalents of sodium each day, and the excretion of sodium must reflect this intake rather closely. Otherwise, serious disturbances of the extracellular fluid volume will soon occur. Glomerular filtration pours about 25,000 mEq of sodium (equal to over 1400 g of sodium chloride) per day into the tubules, which must recover almost all of it while allowing just the right bit to escape into the urine. The fact that a number of different mechanisms share this responsibility provides some insurance against disaster, since the malfunction of one mechanism for sodium excretion can be compensated for, at least partially, by other mechanisms.

However, new mechanisms for intrarenal sodium regulation are still being discovered, and previously established explanations are being challenged. In short, this is an area of very active research and considerable controversy, and we are still a long way from a comprehensive understanding of how the whole system works. Perhaps the least confusing approach to our present-day understanding is via the historical route.

CHANGES IN GLOMERULAR FILTRATION RATE

Several decades ago it was recognized that there is often a direct relationship between glomerular filtration rate and renal sodium excretion. Laboratory experiments with animals showed that maneuvers that increase the GFR are likely to be accompanied by increased sodium excretion, while sodium excretion diminishes when GFR falls.

It was also recognized that the increase or decrease in urinary sodium excretion under these circumstances is far less than the increase or decrease in glomerular filtration of sodium. In short, when GFR increases, much of the additional sodium that is filtered gets resorbed by the tubules, so the increase in urinary sodium excretion is relatively small. When GFR decreases (within certain limits), the opposite adjustment takes place. It appears that the percentage of filtered sodium that is resorbed by the tubules remains about the same when GFR rises or falls; this means, of course, that the percentage of filtered sodium that is excreted also remains about the same. This is true only within certain limits and if other factors influencing sodium excretion do not change. This ability to adjust the resorption of sodium to small changes in GFR is known as *glomerulotubular balance* and is thought to reside in the proximal tubule.

Considering the large amount of sodium in glomerular filtrate, glomerulotubular balance can be regarded as a safety mechanism. It protects against the huge fluctuations of sodium excretion that would occur if the tubules did not adjust to changes in GFR. Table 5-1 illustrates the predicted influence of changes in GFR on proximal resorption and urinary excretion of sodium in the presence and absence of glomerulotubular balance. Other factors influencing sodium resorption are assumed to be unchanged. Filtration, proximal resorption and distal delivery from the proximal tubule are expressed in terms of liters of glomerular filtrate or tubular fluid. Note the large fluctuations in distal delivery of tubular fluid in the absence of glomerulotubular balance. The impact on urinary sodium excretion can only be estimated because we do not know exactly how much the distal nephron will compensate for changes in the amount of tubular fluid it receives.

Because of the observed response of sodium excretion to changes in GFR, a response that is reduced but not abolished by glomerulotubular balance, changes in GFR were once thought to be the dominant mechanism in the regulation of sodium excretion. But although changes in GFR can play some role, they fail to account for the regulation of sodium excretion in many circumstances. For instance, a modest increase in sodium intake will lead to a corresponding increase in sodium excretion without any demonstrable change of GFR. And under some experimental circumstances to be described shortly, sodium excretion may increase despite a decrease in GFR.

Table 5-1. Glomerulotubular Balance

	Filtered	Proximal Reabsorption	Distal Delivery	Sodium in Urine
Control	180 liters/day	144 liters/day	36 liters/day	150 mEq/day
Increased GFR				
With G-T balance	190 liters/day	152 liters/day	38 liters/day	↑
Without G-T balance	190 liters/day	144 liters/day	46 liters/day	↑↑↑
Decreased GFR				
With G-T balance	170 liters/day	136 liters/day	34 liters/day	↓
Without G-T balance	170 liters/day	144 liters/day	26 liters/day	↓↓↓

ALDOSTERONE AND THE GREAT ESCAPE

For many years it has been known that a hormone (or hormones) from the adrenal cortex acts on the kidneys to reduce sodium excretion. It was observed that patients or animals with generalized adrenal cortical insufficiency suffer from renal sodium wasting and that this wasting can be corrected by extracts of normal adrenal glands. The hormone responsible for this effect in man has been identified as aldosterone. We know that it acts on the distal nephron to promote tubular resorption of sodium there. (As we shall see in later chapters, it also promotes the secretion of potassium and hydrogen ions.) Several other steroid compounds, such as desoxycorticosterone (DOCA) and 9-alpha-fluorocortisol, appear to have the same effect; preparations that act in this manner are known as *mineralocorticoid hormones.*

When a mineralocorticoid hormone is administered continuously to a normal subject who is ingesting a significant amount of sodium in the diet, an interesting sequence of events is observed. Sodium virtually disappears from the urine at first and the subject gains weight, reflecting the accumulation of retained sodium and water as additional extracellular fluid. But this process does not continue indefinitely. When a certain amount of fluid has been added, usually several kilograms in a human, sodium reappears in the urine and no further accumulation occurs, despite the continued administration of the mineralocorticoid hormone (Fig. 5-1). This so-called "escape phenomenon" usually takes place before enough additional extracellular fluid has been formed to produce visible edema.

The ability of normal subjects to escape from the sodium-retaining effect of mineralocorticoids shows that these hormones do not have total control of sodium excretion. There must be other mechanisms that, in response to expansion of the extracellular fluid volume, are able to override the sodium-retaining effect of the mineralocorticoids. Another piece of evidence against a dominant role for these hormones is their slow onset of action. It takes nearly an hour for mineralocorticoids to have an effect on renal sodium excretion, but the kidneys can respond much faster to acute reduction of the circulating or extracellular fluid volume.

THE BRITISH BREAKTHROUGH

A now famous experiment performed in 1961 by de Wardener and his colleagues in England and subsequently repeated in other laboratories showed convincingly that glomerular filtration rate and adrenal hormones are not the only factors that control renal sodium excretion. Glomerular filtration rate and renal sodium excretion were measured continuously in a dog given large amounts of a mineralocorticoid hormone before and during the experiment; saline solution was then given intravenously. This caused an escape from the mineralocorticoid effect and the appearance of much sodium in the

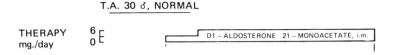

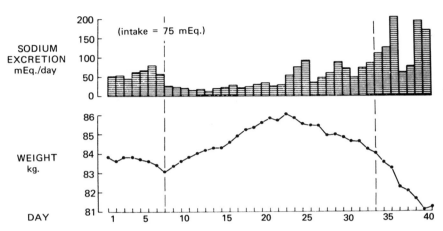

Figure 5-1. Weight gain and temporary reduction of sodium excretion produced by administration of aldosterone to a normal subject on a constant sodium intake. Note the increase of sodium excretion on day 23 (the sixteenth day of aldosterone treatment) despite continued administration of the hormone. (Modified slightly from J. T. August, D. H. Nelson, and G. W. Thorn, *J. Clin. Invest.* 37: 1551, 1958.)

urine. Then, while the saline infusion was continued, the glomerular filtration rate was reduced by inflating a balloon that had previously been placed in the aorta above the renal arteries. Despite this decrease in GFR, renal sodium excretion remained well above that of the baseline period. A similar experiment from another laboratory is illustrated in Figure 5-2.

How did the kidneys know that the extracellular fluid volume had been expanded and that sodium should be excreted, and what intrarenal mechanism accomplished the excretion of sodium? Clearly an increase in glomerular filtration rate (factor 1) was not responsible, since GFR had actually been reduced during the critical period. A decrease in the level of mineralocorticoid hormones (factor 2) was not responsible either, since these had been maintained artificially at supraphysiological levels throughout the experiment. So there must have been something else. The "something else" was referred to in the physiological literature of the time as "third factor." Now, after 20 years and an enormous amount of investigation, it appears that a number of mechanisms may contribute to what was called third factor. There is still no widespread agreement on just how many mechanisms there are and

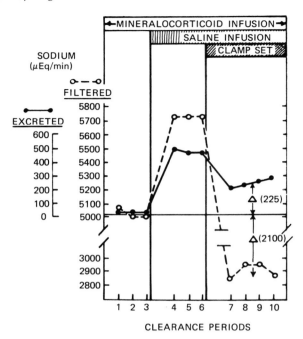

Figure 5-2. Results from a study like the de Wardener experiment described in the text. This work was performed by N. G. Levinsky and reported in *Ann. N.Y. Acad. Sci.* 139: 295, 1966. This investigator tightened a clamp around the aorta above the renal arteries to reduce GFR. The dashed line showing filtered sodium reflects GFR. Note that in the final phase of the study (periods 7 through 10) sodium excretion was greater than in the baseline periods (1 through 3) by 225 μEq/min, even though a fall of GFR had reduced filtered sodium by 2100 μEq/min.

whether some of those suggested even exist, but we shall describe the most promising contenders.

STARLING FORCES IN PERITUBULAR CAPILLARIES

To understand this mechanism, we'll have to look a bit more closely at how sodium is reabsorbed in the proximal tubule. As diagrammed in Figure 5-3, a proximal tubule cell is not uniform on all sides. On one side it has the brush border, composed of many microvilli that project into the tubular lumen. The opposite side of the cell appears to be separated by a small interstitial space from the basement membrane and, beyond that, a peritubular capillary. Electron micrographs show that there are also intercellular channels between the proximal tubular cells and that these connect with the interstitial space at the base of the cells. The intercellular channels are probably not open (at least

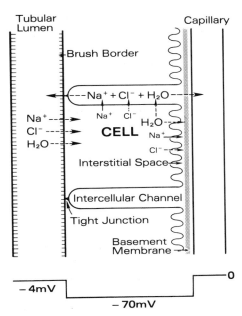

Figure 5-3. Diagram of a proximal tubular cell to show movements of sodium, chloride, and water. Solid arrows represent active transport; dashed arrows represent passive movement. The electrical potentials of the tubular lumen and the cell interior are shown graphically in millivolts (mV). The peritubular capillary is assumed to have a potential of zero.

not all the time) all the way to the tubular lumen; apposition of the cells seems to close them off just short of the lumen. The place where proximal tubular cells come together to close off the intercellular space is referred to as the *tight junction.*

Sodium ions from the tubular lumen diffuse passively through the brush border into the proximal tubular cells in response to electrical and chemical forces, since the interior of the cell is negative with respect to the lumen, and the intracellular concentration of sodium is very low. It is kept that way because pumps at the other borders of the cell extrude sodium actively against a concentration gradient into the interstitial and intercellular spaces. Chloride ions probably follow the same route as the sodium ions from the tubular lumen through the tubular cell to the peritubular fluid, but their movement is believed to be entirely passive in response to forces created by the active movement of sodium. (If chloride or some other anion did not move with sodium, an electrical imbalance would soon develop that would halt the movement of sodium.) The movement of many sodium and chloride ions from the tubular lumen to the other side of the cell would cause the tubular fluid to become hypo-osmotic and the interstitial fluid hyperosmotic, except for the fact that the proximal tubule is very permeable to water. Thus water also moves from the tubular fluid to the peritubular spaces in response to osmotic forces set up by the movement of sodium and chloride. The result of these combined processes is large-scale transfer of sodium, chloride, and water in the same proportions from tubular lumen to spaces on the other side of the proximal tubular cells.

What happens to the accumulating extracellular fluid around the proximal tabules? Obviously it must be collected by the peritubular capillaries and returned to the general circulation. The efficiency with which this process takes place seems to depend on the Starling forces—oncotic and hydrostatic pressures—in the peritubular capillaries. (See Chapter 1 if you don't understand Starling forces.) If the albumin concentration in these capillaries is high and the hydrostatic pressure low, peritubular fluid is picked up efficiently, and relatively little accumulates around the tubular cells. But if capillary albumin concentration is low or hydrostatic pressure high or both, peritubular fluid is not removed efficiently and accumulates around and between the proximal tubular cells. Here it may interfere with the further transport of sodium, chloride, and water across the cells to the peritubular space. According to one plausible explanation, the accumulation of fluid between the cells may force open the tight junction, allowing reabsorbed fluid and electrolytes to leak back into the lumen. (This is known as the pump-leak theory.) Either process—inhibition of further transport or back-leak—can be expected to reduce the overall efficiency of resorption of tubular fluid.

Thanks to some pretty fancy micropuncture work, these nice theories are backed up by experimental evidence. Most of the relevant laboratory studies indicate that there is indeed a positive relationship between albumin concentration in peritubular capillaries and the efficiency of sodium-chloride-water resorption in the proximal tubules. The capillary hydrostatic pressure appears to have the predicted influence also; that is, elevation of pressure in the peritubular capillaries appears to inhibit sodium resorption in the proximal tubules. So most investigators now agree that changes in the peritubular Starling forces are an important mechanism for sodium retrieval by the proximal tubules. We must point out, however, that not all authorities share this view, and there are some experimental results that do not support it.

This still leaves us with the question of what regulates the Starling forces. One obvious determinant is the filtration fraction—the proportion of renal plasma flow filtered by glomeruli. As you know, the process of glomerular filtration removes plasma water from the glomerular capillaries while leaving plasma proteins behind. This raises the concentration of albumin and other proteins in glomerular blood by 20% or more under normal conditions. If the filtration fraction increases, albumin concentration in glomerular efferent blood is raised even more. When you recall that the efferent arterioles from the glomeruli supply the peritubular capillaries, the close relationship between filtration fraction and protein concentration in the peritubular capillaries is apparent. This relationship provides at least a partial explanation for glomerulotubular balance. An increase in filtration fraction generates more tubular fluid (assuming no change in renal blood flow), but it also results in higher peritubular protein concentration that will facilitate retrieval of the additional filtrate from the proximal tubules.

The filtration fraction appears to be regulated largely by hemodynamic factors—the arterial blood pressure supplied to the kidney and the constriction or relaxation of afferent and efferent arterioles. These factors also determine how much hydrostatic pressure will be transmitted to the peritubular capillaries. So it appears that both the oncotic and hydrostatic pressure in these capillaries are under hemodynamic control.

The role of the peritubular Starling forces in the maintenance of glomerulotubular balance seems fairly clear and logical. But glomerulotubular balance, after all, is simply an internal regulation within the kidney which adjusts proximal resorption to changes in GFR. Do Starling forces also play a part in adjusting renal sodium excretion in response to conditions beyond the kidney, such as expansion of the extracellular fluid volume? And if so, how do such influences bring about changes in peritubular oncotic and/or hydrostatic pressures? We do not have clear answers at present, and the explanations proposed get quite complicated. Rather than launch into several pages of murky discussion, we'll leave these questions for the curious reader to pursue in the detailed reviews available elsewhere.

NATRIURETIC HORMONE

As indicated by the de Wardener experiment described earlier in this chapter, the kidneys may respond appropriately to an intravenous saline load even though the glomerular filtration rate is artificially reduced and mineralocorticoid hormones are administered in excess. What signal tells them to excrete sodium?

One attractive explanation is that a *natriuretic hormone* produced somewhere in the body in response to expansion of the extracellular fluid volume acts on the renal tubules to inhibit sodium resorption. Some experimental work appears to support this concept. In one such study, two dogs were connected in a cross-circulation arrangement (Fig. 5-4). Blood was exchanged between the dogs, but a pump between them ensured that the transfer of blood was equal in both directions; that is, there was no net gain or loss of blood by either dog. When saline was infused into one dog, that dog responded as expected with increased sodium excretion. But the other dog, which did not receive a saline infusion, also had a significant though lesser increase of sodium excretion. It was suggested that the dog receiving the saline had produced a circulating natriuretic hormone that acted also on the kidneys of the noninfused dog. Other ingenious experiments have suggested the presence of such a hormone in volume-expanded subjects or those with advanced renal insufficiency, who excrete a relatively high percentage of their filtered sodium.

The trouble is that some other experiments have failed to demonstrate a

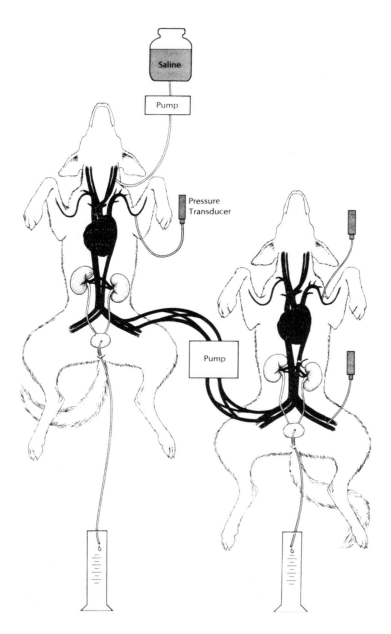

Figure 5-4. Cross-circulation experiment described in the text. (Figure by R. Ingle is reproduced with permission from an article by J. O. Davis in *Hosp. Prac.* 5: 74, October 1970.)

natriuretic hormone. And determined efforts to isolate and purify the hormone have met with limited success. One group of investigators thought they had captured it, but when they took it to another institution for a demonstration, it didn't work. Different laboratories working to isolate the hormone have published differing descriptions of its physical and chemical characteristics. Of course, there could conceivably be more than one natriuretic hormone.

As things stand now, the possible existence of a natriuretic hormone must be regarded as an unresolved issue. Investigation goes on, and its believers and nonbelievers continue to debate the question fervently.

REDISTRIBUTION OF RENAL BLOOD FLOW

It has long been recognized that there are anatomical differences between nephrons. In particular, nephrons which are located deep in the cortex near the corticomedullary junction (the so-called *juxtamedullary nephrons*) differ as a group from more superficial nephrons. Compared with superficial nephrons, juxtamedullary nephrons have larger glomeruli and longer tubules. Their loops of Henle extend deep into the medulla and in some cases to the tips of the renal papillae. In contrast, superficial nephrons have attenuated loops of Henle which extend only a short distance into the medulla and in some cases do not even leave the cortex.

Despite their larger glomeruli and presumed greater filtering ability, it has been postulated that the juxtamedullary nephrons are better designed than superficial nephrons for the efficient resorption of sodium because of their long tubular system. This hypothesis cannot be examined directly by micropuncture studies because the renal cortical surface contains only the proximal and distal convoluted tubules of *superficial* nephrons. Loops of Henle have been studied by micropuncture at the tips of renal papillae, but only the loops of *deep* nephrons are found there. It is difficult to make valid comparisons between the two types of nephrons when comparable parts of these nephrons cannot be studied. So the premise that juxtamedullary nephrons reabsorb sodium more efficiently than superficial nephrons rests on indirect evidence only and is far from established.

Some experimental evidence suggests that conditions associated with renal sodium retention, such as real or apparent depletion of circulatory volume, are associated with a marked reduction of blood flow to the superficial renal cortex, while the deep cortex and medullary regions seem to be less affected. This led to the hypothesis that one mechanism for renal sodium regulation might be a shifting of blood flow between superficial salt-losing nephrons and deep salt-retaining nephrons. Other laboratory work using different methods does not support this view, however, and most authorities at present do not feel that this is a significant mechanism for regulation of sodium excretion.

OTHER FACTORS

The renal nerves or circulating catecholamines or both may influence renal sodium excretion. Stimulation of the renal nerves decreases the sodium content of the urine, while denervation of one kidney is followed by greater sodium output from that kidney. It is easy to suppose that such maneuvers might affect sodium excretion through an effect on renal hemodynamics by causing constriction or relaxation of afferent or efferent arterioles. Yet there is also some anatomical and physiological evidence to suggest that renal nerves innervate renal tubules and stimulate them to reabsorb sodium. We have no idea how this works at the cellular level—if indeed it is a real phenomenon. Since transplanted kidneys, which are denervated, can conserve or excrete sodium appropriately, the importance of the renal nerves in regulating sodium excretion under normal circumstances remains in some doubt.

Prostaglandins and elements of the kallikrein-kinin system are also present in the kidney. Under some conditions these vasoactive substances appear to influence a number of renal functions, including sodium excretion. Although these hormones could eventually prove to be of considerable importance, their normal physiological roles in the kidney are not clear at the present time.

PERSPECTIVE

The enormous resorption of sodium that takes place in the proximal tubules ensures the recovery of most of the glomerular filtrate and smooths out the delivery of electrolyte and filtrate to the distal parts of the nephrons. Not too many years ago it was believed that small adjustments in sodium excretion were achieved by changes in proximal sodium resorption. Now it is generally felt that the proximal tubules do a bulk-processing job and that the fine regulation of sodium excretion takes place farther downstream in the tubules. For instance, small changes in sodium intake appear to have no effect on sodium resorption in the proximal tubules, though they result in appropriate changes in sodium excretion; the distal parts of the nephrons must be making the adjustments by mechanisms we don't understand at present.

When large changes in sodium excretion are called for, however, the proximal tubules apparently do play a role in the regulation. Marked expansion of the extracellular fluid volume causes a demonstrable decrease in proximal sodium resorption with a significant increase in delivery of fluid and electrolyte to the distal nephrons. Conversely, a decrease in extracellular fluid volume, which need not be of impressive proportions, appears to enhance proximal sodium resorption and reduce distal delivery. This can have important consequences in some clinical situations.

Obviously, there are still gaps in our knowledge about the renal mechanisms of sodium resorption. Though some of these mechanisms have been identified, there are surely still others waiting to be discovered. A comprehensive understanding of the process will have to wait for future insights.

BIBLIOGRAPHY

S. Klahr and E. Slatopolsky. Renal regulation of sodium excretion. Function in health and edema-forming states. *Arch. Intern. Med.* 131: 780–791, 1973.

H. E. de Wardener. The control of sodium excretion. *Am. J. Physiol.* 235: F163–F173, 1978.

6
How the Kidneys Regulate Water Excretion

In Chapter 4 we learned that renal excretion or conservation of water is governed under normal circumstances by the osmolality and sometimes the effective volume of the serum and extracellular fluid. A low serum osmolality promotes the renal excretion of water—especially if extracellular fluid volume is normal or high—and this has the effect of raising serum osmolality toward normal. High serum osmolality or contraction of extracellular fluid volume inhibits the renal excretion of water; unnecessary losses of water under such circumstances would make matters worse. An important part of the effector system for these adjustments is vasopressin, the antidiuretic hormone (ADH), whose presence or absence largely determines how much water the urine will contain, that is, whether the urine will be concentrated or dilute. Our purpose in this chapter is to examine the mechanisms within the kidney that enable it to produce either concentrated or dilute urine as the need arises.

We may think of urine as having two major components, solute and water. Quantitatively the most important solutes in urine are urea and the salts of sodium and potassium; the amounts that need to be excreted in order to maintain internal homeostasis will normally depend on the dietary intake of nitrogen, sodium, and potassium. Eating habits vary considerably between individuals, of course, but a person on a typical American diet might excrete about 900 mOsm of solute each day. Given this amount of solute as an excretory obligation, the kidneys can vary the amount of water lost with it over a wide range, producing urine that may have an osmolality as high as 1200 mOsm/kg water or more, or as low as 100 mOsm/kg water or less.*

These changes in urine concentration have a profound effect on urine volume and thus on the conservation or excretion of water. Table 6-1 gives

---

*As explained in Chapter 1, the osmolality of a solution is expressed as milliosmoles per kilogram of water (mOsm/kg water). This is a cumbersome expression to use repeatedly, however, and so for the remainder of this chapter we shall shorten it to simply "mOsm."

Table 6-1. Alternative Ways of Excreting 900 mOsm/Day

Urine Osm (mOsm/kg)	Urine Volume (ml/day)	Water Saved (+) or Lost (−)[a]
100	9000	−6000
150	6000	−3000
300	3000	
600	1500	+1500
900	1000	+2000
1200	750	+2250

[a]Additional milliliters per day retained (+) or excreted (−) when compared with water excretion at urine osmolality of 300 mOsm/kg.

some illustrative numbers. Figures are given for urine volumes that will result if the same osmolar load—900 mOsm in this case—is excreted at osmolalities ranging from 100 to 1200 mOsm. The column on the right shows the additional water that is lost (−) or retained (+) by the body at each osmolality when compared with the water loss at a urine concentration of 300 mOsm, which is approximately isotonic with plasma. While a significant amount of water may be conserved by producing a concentrated (hypertonic) urine, it pales by comparison with the additional water that may be excreted by producing a dilute (hypotonic) urine. This flexibility of water excretion gives us and other land mammals a great deal of freedom—freedom from the need to match water intake closely to physiological requirements. Thanks to our kidneys, we can drink any reasonable amount of fluid without risk of internal disaster.

The loop of Henle, which makes possible the production of hypertonic urine, was regarded as an anatomical curiosity until little more than thirty years ago. Why should some renal tubules make a long detour into the renal medulla and back before joining a collecting duct? It had indeed been recognized by some investigators that there was generally a relationship between the length of Henle's loop in an animal species and the ability of that species to produce a hypertonic urine: The longer the loop, the more concentrated the urine that could be formed. But the reasons for this relationship remained elusive until the 1940s when Kuhn and his coworkers proposed the *countercurrent hypothesis*. Their theory stood the test of numerous laboratory studies and gained general acceptance in the 1960s. Their explanation of the workings of Henle's loop, now called the countercurrent *mechanism* in keeping with its "established" status, seems so logical that you may wonder why no one thought of it sooner.

THE MAJORITY VIEW

There is still debate about some of the details of the countercurrent mechanism. The account here will describe the view of most renal physiologists with occasional references to alternative explanations. Let's look at the system by following tubular fluid through the nephron (Fig. 6-1).

As described in Chapter 2, most of the glomerular filtrate is reabsorbed in the proximal tubule. Due to the water-permeable nature of the proximal tubule, its fluid remains virtually isotonic with plasma water. The concentration of sodium does not change significantly from the beginning to the end of the proximal tubule, though there is much less of both sodium and water at the end.

The isotonic fluid at the end of the proximal tubule then empties into the descending limb of Henle's loop, which is also permeable to water and probably to small solutes as well. But unlike the proximal tubule, which is sur-

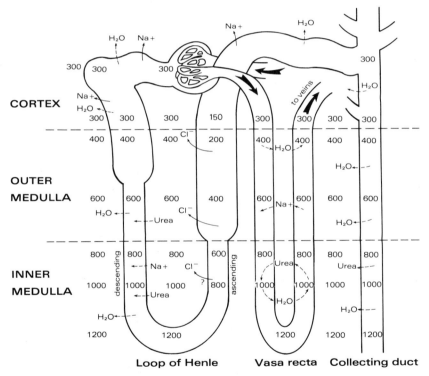

Figure 6-1. Diagram of a juxtamedullary nephron showing osmotic changes as fluid passes through the tubule during production of hypertonic urine. Numbers show the approximate osmolality of tubular fluid or interstitial tissue in milliosmols per kilogram of water. Active transport of sodium or chloride is shown by solid arrows; passive movement of sodium, chloride, water, or urea by dashed arrows. Since electrical balance must be maintained, the movements shown for sodium are accompanied by an anion (usually chloride), and those shown for chloride are accompanied by a cation (usually sodium). A vascular loop is also shown to demonstrate osmotic changes in the vasa recta.

rounded in the renal cortex by tissue that is isotonic with plasma, the descending limb of Henle's loop passes through medullary tissue that becomes increasingly hypertonic as the renal papilla is approached. The hypertonicity is due principally to the high concentrations of sodium, chloride, and urea in the medullary tissue. Since the descending limb is permeable, its tubular fluid tends to equilibrate with the osmolality of the surrounding tissue. Some investigators believe that this osmotic equilibration is accomplished almost entirely by the loss of water from the tubular fluid to the medullary interstitium; others stress the entrance of sodium, chloride, and urea into the tubular fluid from the interstitium. It seems likely that both of these processes have a significant role.

At the tip or "hairpin turn" of a long loop of Henle, the tubular fluid in a human kidney may have an osmolality of 1200 mOsm or higher. This is about four times the osmolality of glomerular filtrate.

On rounding the hairpin turn, our tubular fluid enters the ascending limb of Henle's loop, which differs markedly from the descending limb in structure and function. For one thing, the ascending limb is relatively impermeable even to water. For another, it is a site of active transport rather than passive diffusion. As tubular fluid moves back toward the cortex, the cells of the ascending limb transport chloride ions out of the fluid and into the medullary interstitium. Sodium follows in response to electrical forces set up by the transport of chloride. Water *cannot* follow osmotically, however, because the ascending limb isn't permeable to it. So the tubular fluid in the ascending limb becomes hypotonic to the surrounding tissue, and the medullary interstitium is rendered more hypertonic by the transfer of chloride and sodium. In fact, it is this active transport of chloride by the ascending limb that maintains the renal medulla in its hypertonic state.

(Until a few years ago it was believed that sodium was transported actively in the ascending limb, with the chloride going along passively, and this version of the process is still found in many books. For our purposes it doesn't much matter, since the end result—transfer of sodium and chloride—is the same.)

As tubular fluid passes up the ascending limb, its osmolality decreases progressively as more and more chloride and sodium are removed from it. The osmotic gradient between the tubular fluid and the interstitium would thus become greater and greater—except for the fact that the osmolality of the surrounding interstitium is also decreasing as the tubule approaches the renal cortex. Thus the osmotic gap between the inside and the outside of the ascending limb remains about the same all the way up to the cortex even though both osmolalities are decreasing progressively. And when the ascending limb reaches the cortex, which is not hypertonic, its tubular fluid is actually dilute compared to plasma. This hypotonic fluid enters the distal convoluted tubule.

The events described thus far are the same regardless of whether concentrated or dilute urine is to be formed eventually. The final creation of hypertonic or hypotonic urine depends on events beyond the loop of Henle.

If the body requires water conservation and the production of hypertonic urine, vasopressin is liberated into the bloodstream. In response to this hormone the collecting duct and probably at least part of the distal convoluted tubule both become permeable to water. Since the fluid that the distal convoluted tubule receives from Henle's loop is hypotonic, water diffuses out of the permeable part of the distal tubule and the cortical part of the collecting duct until the osmolality of the tubular fluid rises to that of the surrounding cortex. The tubular fluid is now back to the osmolality of the original glomerular filtrate.

In the collecting duct the tubular fluid must pass once more through the renal medulla, which becomes increasingly hypertonic as the renal pelvis is approached. Because the vasopressin-sensitive collecting duct is permeable, tubular water diffuses from it into the medullary interstitium, raising the osmolality of the remaining tubular fluid. The final product, urine, can have an osmolality that closely approaches that of the tip of the renal medulla.

Vasopressin also increases the permeability of the collecting duct to urea. Since urea diffuses from the permeable portions of the nephron less easily than water, it becomes concentrated to some extent on the way through the nephron and quite concentrated in the collecting duct. Because of this high concentration in the collecting duct and the vasopressin-induced permeability there, a significant amount of urea diffuses from the collecting duct into the medullary interstitium of the concentrating kidney, contributing to the high osmolality of the medulla. The immediate effect, at least, is to permit the removal of more water from the urine, though at the expense of excreting less urea.

If a dilute urine is to be produced, the events we have described in the loop of Henle remain the same qualitatively, though the osmolality in the medulla may be less than in the concentrating kidney. But a major difference is found in the vasopressin-sensitive parts of the nephron. Vasopressin is no longer present, and in its absence the entire distal nephron remains relatively impermeable to water. So the hypotonic fluid that emerges from the ascending limb of Henle's loop does not equilibrate osmotically with the surrounding tissue. It remains hypotonic as it passes through the late portions of the nephron and the collecting duct; it may, in fact, become more hypotonic because of further resorption of sodium from the lumen in the distal convoluted tubule and collecting duct. The result is the delivery of hypotonic fluid (i.e., dilute urine) to the renal pelvis.

Thus the permeability changes induced in the distal nephron by vasopressin or its lack can make the difference between a meager amount of concentrated urine and a generous flood of very watery urine.

AN ALTERNATIVE EXPLANATION

The appearance of the cells in the first part of the ascending limb (the *thin* ascending limb of Henle's loop) is puzzling and disturbing to thoughtful physiologists. In contrast to the robust-looking cells of the thick ascending limb that follows, the cells of the thin ascending limb look puny and poorly suited for the heavy work of transporting chloride out of the lumen against a gradient. Physiologists have tried to figure out how the system might work if these cells in fact do not engage in active transport. One explanation, suggested with some experimental support, is that the descending limb of Henle's loop might be almost impermeable to small solutes, though quite permeable to water. Sodium and chloride in the descending limb would then become so concentrated by the removal of water that they could diffuse *passively* (or be transported with minimal work) from the thin ascending limb into the interstitium, where their concentration is lower. According to this view, urea would not diffuse into the descending limb. Its high concentration in the medullary interstitium would provide much of the osmotic force needed to remove water from the descending limb and thus raise the chloride and sodium concentrations there above their concentrations in the interstitium. It is an interesting and controversial idea. At least everyone seems to agree that active transport of chloride takes place from the *thick* ascending limb of Henle's loop.

One important aspect of this system is the arrangement of the blood vessels in the medulla. As mentioned in Chapter 2, efferent arterioles from juxtamedullary glomeruli give rise to long capillary loops, the vasa recta, which dip into the medulla and then return to the cortex, a round trip that takes them through a hyperosmotic area. Since these capillary loops are permeable to water and small molecules, the blood in them loses water and takes up solute as it descends into the hypertonic medulla, a process that tends to dilute the osmolality there (Fig. 6-1). But the process is reversed on the return trip to the cortex. As the now-hypertonic blood enters areas of decreasing osmolality, it loses solute to the interstitium and takes back water from it, thus repairing much of the osmotic damage done on the downward trip. This arrangement, called a *countercurrent exchange* mechanism, helps to minimize the net loss of osmolality caused by the flow of blood through the renal medulla.

SOME QUESTIONS AND ANSWERS

At this point we shall try to answer some of the most-asked questions about the renal concentrating-diluting mechanism.

Question

How does the osmotic gradient in the renal medulla get established in the first place?

Answer

That's difficult to explain without a diagram—see Figure 6-2, which represents the descending and ascending limbs of Henle's loop and the renal medullary tissue, or interstitium, between them. (We left out the collecting

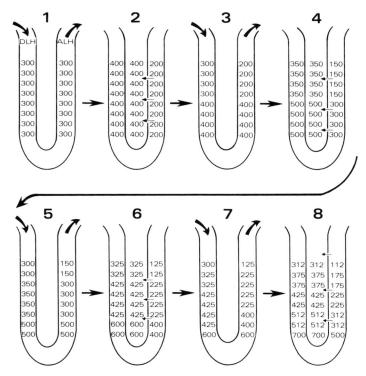

Figure 6-2. Scheme to show how an osmotic gradient might be generated in the medullary interstitium by the loop of Henle. The sequence of events is explained in the text. DLH = descending limb of Henle's loop. ALH = ascending limb of Henle's loop. (Redrawn and modified with permission from R. F. Pitts, *Physiology of the Kidney and Body Fluids*, 3rd ed., Year Book Medical Publishers, Chicago, 1974.)

duct and vasa recta because we don't need them right now.) Flow of tubular fluid through the loop of Henle is shown in odd-numbered frames, and the action of chloride pumps in even-numbered frames, although both processes actually occur simultaneously.

Let's start with the whole system at the osmolality of plasma water, approximately 300 mOsm (frame 1). Now picture the ascending limb of Henle's loop as being able to generate a limited osmotic gradient of about 200 mOsm between its lumen and the interstitium by pumping out chloride. This raises the osmolality of the medullary interstitium and thus the osmolality in the descending limb, which equilibrates osmotically with it (frame 2). The fluid that now comes around the hairpin turn into the ascending limb has a higher osmolality than previously (frame 3), thus enabling the cells of the ascending limb to pump more solute into the interstitium (frame 4). This raises the osmolality of the interstitium and the descending limb still further, and the same sequence of events is repeated over and over. Thus, the so-called *single effect* (the ability of a tubular cell to create a limited osmotic gradient by active transport) can be multiplied many times by the movement of tubular fluid and the arrangement of the loops until a large osmolality is built up at the tip of the medulla.

Question

The ascending limb of Henle's loop is pumping chloride and sodium into the medulla to make it hypertonic, but water diffusing from the collecting duct must be diluting the medulla. Don't these two processes neutralize each other? How can the medulla remain hypertonic under these circumstances?

Answer

Water from the collecting ducts does indeed dilute the medulla, but there is relatively more solute being removed from Henle's ascending limbs than there is water coming from the collecting ducts. How can this be if the final urine is hypertonic? The answer is that, when concentrated urine is being formed, most of the extra water that must be removed from the tubular fluid gets dumped in the renal cortex where there is no osmotic gradient to protect.

A matter of simple arithmetic: In round numbers, suppose that the hypotonic tubular fluid that reaches the cortex from the ascending limb of Henle's loop has an osmolality of 150 mOsm. Osmotic equilibration in the distal convoluted tubule and the cortical part of the collecting duct will raise this osmolality to about 300 mOsm. If the amount of solute in the tubules remained the same, removal of 50% of the water would be required in order to double the osmolality. Since some net resorption of solute is taking place in this part of the nephron, even more than 50% of the water in the tubular fluid must be removed in order to raise its osmolality to 300 mOsm. So most of the water delivered from the loop of Henle never reaches the medullary part of the collecting duct. Even if 75% of the remaining water must be removed by the medullary collecting duct in order to raise the urine to 1200 mOsm, this is now a relatively small amount of water.

Question

What happens to the water that enters the medullary interstitium from the collecting duct?

Answer

It is carried back into the circulation by the ascending vasa recta. When you think about it, that is what *has* to happen. There are five types of tubes passing through the medulla. Three of them—the descending limbs of Henle's loops, the collecting ducts, and the descending vasa recta—deliver water *to* the medulla because of osmotic gradients; the ascending limbs of Henle's loops, another type, are impermeable. Since the medulla doesn't appear to have lymphatic drainage, that leaves the ascending vasa recta to carry away the water; this must be happening, since the renal medulla doesn't swell up and burst. The water is removed along with solutes from which it cannot be separated in the interstitium of the medulla.

Question

How can urine of intermediate osmolality (neither maximally concentrated nor maximally diluted) be produced?

Answer

Although we have talked about vasopressin as being either present or absent, its release into the circulation is not really an all-or-nothing phenomenon. Depending on the situation, it can be released rapidly or slowly to produce a spectrum of serum concentrations. And in response to those differing serum concentrations of vasopressin, the permeability of sensitive portions of the nephron may vary over a wide range. When the distal nephron is only partially permeable to water, osmotic equilibration between tubular fluid and the surrounding renal tissue will be incomplete, resulting in the production of urine with intermediate osmolality. Except under physiologically stressful circumstances, such as water deprivation, human urine is generally of intermediate osmolality, often moderately hypertonic to plasma.

Question

Some nephrons have very short loops of Henle. Can these nephrons produce hypertonic urine?

Answer

Yes—with help. The collecting ducts are the final common pathway through which tubular fluid from all nephrons must pass before leaving the kidney. All collecting ducts must traverse the full thickness of the medulla in order to reach the renal pelvis. So in its final passage tubular fluid from all nephrons, even those with short loops, can be exposed to high medullary osmolalities and made hypertonic.

Of course, not all nephrons are contributing equally to the work of producing hypertonic urine. The whole process depends on those with long loops of Henle which are pumping chloride ions into the interstitium deep in the renal medulla, thus maintaining medullary hypertonicity. The situation might be compared to a subway train made up of similar-looking cars, only some of which have motors; the whole train moves at the same speed, even though some cars are doing all the work! (This comparison applies only to the process of concentrating urine, since there is no reason to believe that nephrons with short loops are getting a free ride in other respects.)

However, the maximum urine osmolality which can be achieved depends on medullary osmolality. This depends, in turn, on the equilibrium that is reached between the continuous active addition of solute to the medulla and the continuous passive erosion of medullary hypertonicity by diffusion, blood flow and the addition of water. The rate at which solute can be added to the medulla is related to the number of nephrons with long loops of Henle. Therefore animals with a high proportion of long loops can generally produce a more concentrated urine that those with fewer long loops.

Question

What does all this countercurrent activity accomplish? Couldn't a simpler system do the job?

Answer

Would nature be stupid enough to build anything this complicated if it didn't accomplish something? Superficially, it might appear easier to form concentrated urine by the active transport (resorption) of water from a straight tubule. But the transport of water, as opposed to the transport of solutes, would require far more energy, and the cells at the distal end of the tubule would have to transport water against a very high osmotic gradient, a difficult if not impossible task.

The countercurrent mechanism is an efficient system that allows the formation of highly concentrated urine without requiring individual cells to transport against an unreasonable osmotic gradient. The necessary osmotic gradient can be achieved by multiplying the limited *single effect* of individual cells, a multiplication made possible by the anatomical relationships in the countercurrent system.

DISTURBANCES OF RENAL WATER REGULATION

It is not appropriate in a book like this to go into detail about all the conditions—and there are quite a few—known to upset renal water regulation. Nevertheless, you should at least be aware of the most important disorders that can interfere with the mechanisms we have been considering. We shall begin with a brief description of some problems directly related to vasopressin and its effects. The best known of these are well-defined abnormalities whose causes and consequences are easy to understand.

Disorders Related to Vasopressin and Its Effect on Tubules

Lack of vasopressin causing diabetes insipidus is a rare but dramatic disorder in which there is a partial or total lack of ability to produce vasopressin. It occurs as an inherited disease but may also appear spontaneously or in association with injuries or tumors that damage the hypothalamus or posterior pituitary. The kidneys are normal. Without the influence of vasopressin their distal convoluted tubules and collecting ducts are always relatively impermeable to water; therefore, the hypotonic fluid emerging from the ascending limbs of Henle's loops does not come into osmotic equilibrium with the surrounding renal tissue either in the cortex or during its passage down the collecting ducts.

The result is copious volumes of dilute urine, similar to what would be produced if a normal person were to suppress his release of vasopressin by drinking large amounts of water all day and all night. It is not unusual for people with diabetes insipidus to excrete 8 to 10 liters daily of urine that looks like water and has an osmolality of 100 mOsm, more or less. This large ongoing loss of water threatens these patients continuously with dehydration. Fortunately, the thirst mechanism comes to their rescue, and if adequate water is available they can preserve internal homeostasis by drinking enough to keep up with the urinary losses. However, the requirement to drink that much fluid and to urinate a great deal may be a significant nuisance that interferes with sleep and other normal activities. And if the patient is deprived of water, or is an infant (who cannot verbalize his thirst), serious dehydration may develop rapidly.

This form of disease is sometimes called *hypothalamic* or *vasopressin-sensitive diabetes insipidus* because administration of vasopressin results in an abrupt reduction or urine volume with a significant rise in osmolality, a response that is useful in establishing a specific diagnosis.

Vasopressin-resistant diabetes insipidus has a different mechanism. Here the distal nephron remains relatively impermeable to water despite the presence of even large amounts of vasopressin. This inability to respond to vasopressin may be inherited, or it may be caused (usually reversibly) by certain drugs, of which lithium is now the most common. In the inherited form of the disease the clinical features are similar to those in vasopressin-sensitive diabetes insipidus—except, of course, for the lack of response to vasopressin. Where the disorder is drug-induced, it is often of lesser severity, since the offending drug may not be present in high enough concentration to block the tubular effect of vasopressin completely. Vasopressin-resistant diabetes insipidus is also called *nephrogenic diabetes insipidus,* reflecting the fact that the concentrating defect is due to renal unresponsiveness rather than to lack of the anti-diuretic hormone.

Inappropriate secretion of vasopressin, sometimes called the *syndrome of inappropriate ADH* or simply SIADH, is the opposite of vasopressin-sensitive diabetes insipidus. Instead of a lack of vasopressin, there is too much. In both conditions the kidneys are normal, the innocent agents of an endocrine disorder arising somewhere else. In the case of inappropriate ADH the culprit is often a malignant tumor that is producing vasopressin or some other substance with a vasopressinlike effect on renal tubules. In this situation production of vasopressin is not controlled by physiological stimuli; it is released into the circulation whether it is needed or not, and it can't be turned off by the mechanisms that inhibit the normal release of vasopressin. Since significant amounts of vasopressin are in the circulation continuously, the distal tubules and collecting ducts remain permeable to water and tend to form a concentrated urine. The osmolality of the urine varies considerably (it may not even be markedly hypertonic) but the important thing is that the kidneys are prevented from forming urine as dilute as the circumstances may require.

If the patient ingests more water than the kidneys can excrete with their limited dilutional abilities, water retention and hyponatremia result. The retained water expands all body compartments, and expansion of the extracellular fluid compartment can be sufficient to trigger the renal excretion of sodium, resulting in substantial urinary sodium losses in the face of hyponatremia. (This provides some of the evidence that the renal excretion of sodium is controlled by the volume of the plasma or extracellular fluid or both, not by the serum sodium concentration.)

Inappropriate secretion of ADH is not always caused by tumors. It is also found in other situations, including nonmalignant lesions in the lungs or central nervous system. Sometimes the normal source of vasopressin—hypothalamus and posterior pituitary—may be responsible for its abnormal release.

A word of caution, though: For a number of years any patient with impaired ability to form dilute urine and resulting hyponatremia was likely to be labeled as having inappropriate ADH secretion. Recently, some authors have argued that many of these patients were releasing vasopressin in response to normal physiological stimuli such as volume depletion and that it was therefore not proper to call this inappropriate. In short, what seems inappropriate in terms of osmotic regulation may be appropriate in terms of protecting body fluid volumes. The purists have their point; perhaps we should reserve the term *inappropriate ADH* for situations where it is clear that there is no physiological stimulus for the release of vasopressin.

Other Influences on Renal Water Excretion

So far we have been talking as though vasopressin is the only variable that determines the concentration or dilution or urine. Vasopressin does indeed appear to be the controlling influence under normal conditions, the regulator of hour-to-hour changes in urine volume in response to a variable intake of water. But some conditions that can be produced in the laboratory and observed in real life make it apparent that other influences may modify the effect of vasopressin on urinary concentration and even override it at times. Here are some examples:

Example

A strain of rats has diabetes insipidus because of an inherited inability to synthesize vasopressin. Normally these animals produce enormous amounts of urine with an osmolality of about 100 mOsm. But if these rats are deprived of water and allowed to become severely dehydrated, the volume of the urine falls drastically, and its osmolality may rise to moderately hypertonic levels.

Comment

These rats don't know how to make vasopressin, but in this situation they can produce hypertonic urine without it. How? The evidence suggests that under these circumstances of severe volume depletion there is a reduction of glomerular filtration rate and an increase in the percentage of filtrate reabsorbed by the proximal tubules. Thus the volume of tubular fluid delivered to the distal nephrons is reduced. Even when there is no vasopressin, the distal convoluted tubule and collecting duct have some permeability to water. This is not noticeable when there is a large volume of fluid flowing through them. But when the tubular fluid is reduced to a trickle, the amount of water reabsorbed at these sites can raise the urine osmolality significantly. (Resorption of a volume of water from a small pool will have more osmotic effect on the remaining pool than would resorption of the same volume of water from a much larger pool.)

Example

Urine is collected independently from the two ureters of an anesthetized dog. The dog is water-loaded to suppress vasopressin release, and dilute urine is observed coming from both kidneys. Now, the blood flow to one kidney is reduced markedly by tightening a stricture around the renal artery. The urine osmolality on that side rises to hypertronic levels, though dilute urine is still being produced by the kidney with normal blood flow. With further constriction of the renal artery, the urine osmolality falls to isotonic. With still further constriction, urine flow ceases.

Comment

The mechanisms at work here are probably similar to those in the preceding example, although the design of the experiment calls attention to the importance of the blood supply to the kidney. Inability to dilute the urine after constriction of the renal artery may be reflecting decreased glomerular filtration rate, increased proximal resorption, and decreased distal delivery of tubular fluid. Inability to concentrate urine after the additional constriction of the renal artery might result from insufficient delivery to the chloride pumps in the ascending limb of Henle's loop, so that medullary hyperosmolality cannot be maintained. With the final constriction glomerular filtration probably ceases.

Example

Superphysiologic doses of vasopressin are given to a subject, causing the urine to become hypertonic. While the action of vasopressin continues, an intravenous infusion of mannitol is started as a hypertonic solution. (Mannitol is a solute filtered by the glomeruli but not reabsorbed by the tubules.) The infusion rate of mannitol is then increased by steps. As increasing quantities of mannitol appear in the urine, urine volume increases and urine osmolality falls progressively despite the continuing influence of exogenous vasopressin. If the load of mannitol in the urine becomes great enough, the urine will become nearly isotonic.

Comment

This phenomenon, called an *osmotic diuresis,* may be observed whenever a large quantity of any solute must be excreted by the kidneys. The presence in the tubules of large numbers of unreabsorbed osmotic particles interferes with the resorption of water and even other solutes. Urinary concentration is impaired by an osmotic diuresis in part because the large quantity of fluid delivered to the collecting duct overwhelms its ability to reabsorb water. Interference with chloride resorption from the ascending limb of Henle's loop is also a factor because it hampers the ability to maintain medullary hyper-tonicity.

From these and other observations it is apparent that vasopressin cannot control renal water excretion by itself. Its ability to regulate urine osmolality depends on the proper function and balance of many factors. Only when these other parts of the system are working normally does vasopressin appear to be in control. Some of the more important influences on the con-centrating-diluting mechanism appear to be:

- *Renal circulation.* This can be disturbed by poor cardiac output, drastic changes in blood pressure or physical interference with the blood vessels.
- *Volume of plasma or extracellular fluid.* Even small reductions may impair renal diluting ability.
- *Osmotic load.* As seen in one of the preceding examples, the need to excrete an excessive amount of osmoles influences urinary concentration (and dilution at times). A common clinical example of osmotic diuresis is seen in patients with poorly controlled diabetes mellitus who have large amounts of unreabsorbed glucose in their tubular fluid and urine.
- *Hormones.* Adrenal cortical hormones are necessary for adequate urinary dilution; thyroid hormones may be also. Catecholamines may have an influence on urinary concentration, and intrarenal prostaglandins may mediate the effects of other hormones. Except for the adrenal cortical hormones, whose significant permissive role in urinary dilution has been knwon for a long time, the clinical importance of hormones other than vasopressin in urinary concentration and dilution remains uncertain, though new interactions are reported from the laboratory every year.
- *Renal structural integrity.* Diseases that disrupt anatomical relationships, especially in the renal medulla, can interfere with urinary concentration.
- *Chemical disturbances.* Hypercalcemia and hypokalemia have both been asso-ciated with impaired ability to concentrate urine.

• *Drugs.* The list is long, but the most important group to remember is the diuretics.

Many of these influences overlap with each other. For example, a lack of adrenal cortical hormones may result in extracellular fluid volume depletion and circulatory changes; diuretic drugs increase the osmotic load to the tubules. Although most of these influences are independent of vasopressin, some may also affect its release or its action at the cellular level. Depletion of the extracellular fluid volume, for example, triggers the release of vasopressin in addition to having independent effects on renal tubular resorption.

We shall not attempt a more lengthy discussion of these various influences on renal water excretion with their mechanisms and interactions. The reader may already feel considerable confusion—in company with many professionals in this complex field. It is reassuring to remember, however, that the renal process of concentrating or diluting the urine consists of only a few essential steps:

1. The proximal tubule must deliver a proper amount of tubular fluid to the distal nephron.
2. Electrolyte pumps in the ascending limb of Henle's loop act on this fluid, rendering it hypotonic and building a hypertonic environment in the renal medulla.
3. Additional electrolyte pumps in the distal convoluted tubule and collecting duct aid in forming hypotonic urine.
4. The final osmolality of the urine is determined in the distal tubule and collecting duct and is usually controlled by their permeability.
5. That permeability is determined primarily by the presence or absence of vasopressin and the responsiveness of the distal tubules and collecting ducts to it.

All of the other influences we have mentioned must act by affecting one or more of these steps. It is easier and more satisfactory to think in terms of physiological mechanisms that may be disturbed than to memorize all the specific conditions that may interfere with them.

BIBLIOGRAPHY

T. P. Dousa and H. Valtin. Cellular actions of vasopressin in the mammalian kidney. *Kidney Int.* 10: 46–63, 1976.

Some other articles in the same issue of Kidney International *also deal with aspects of renal water regulation.*

J. T. Harrington and J. J. Cohen. Clinical disorders of urine concentration and dilution. *Arch. Intern. Med.* 141: 810–825, 1973.

J. P. Kokko. Renal concentrating and diluting mechanisms. *Hosp. Prac.* 14: 110–116, February, 1979.

> *A readable but sophisticated review of the concentrating mechanism. Dr. Kokko is the major proponent of the theory that sodium and chloride diffuse passively from the thin ascending limb of Henle's loop, and this discussion reflects that point of view.*

R. W. Schrier and T. Berl. Nonosmolar factors affecting renal water excretion. *N. Engl. J. Med.* 292: 81–88 and 141–145, 1975.

7
How the Kidneys
Regulate Hydrogen Ion

THE DIMENSIONS OF THE PROBLEM

The hydrogen ion (H^+) concentration of the internal environment must be held within a certain range if cells are to survive and function. Human plasma normally has a pH between 7.35 and 7.45, while variations between 7.10 and 7.70 may be seen with diseases that upset acid-base balance. Variations beyond this latter range occur only with very severe illnesses and are considered to be life threatening, though quite a few patients with a pH less than 7.0 have survived.

These figures suggest that only slight variations in hydrogen ion concentration are tolerable. However, if we translate the logarithmic pH scale into mEq/liter, we see that:

$$pH \ 7.1 = 0.00008 \ mEq/liter \ of \ H^+$$
$$pH \ 7.4 = 0.00004 \ mEq/liter \ of \ H^+$$
$$pH \ 7.7 = 0.00002 \ mEq/liter \ of \ H^+$$

Thus the cells can withstand at least a fourfold variation in the H^+ concentration of the internal environment.

On the other hand, the absolute amount of H^+ present is minute in comparison with major plasma electrolytes. Hydrogen ion concentration is about 0.0000003 that of sodium, for instance. Seen in these terms, free hydrogen ion is a substance so potent that very small amounts of it can cause disastrous internal pollution.

Now consider the fact that 13,000 mEq of potential H^+ enters the system each day as CO_2, and about 70 mEq more as acid-forming substances in the average American diet. If even the latter amount of free hydrogen ion were added to 42 liters of pure water, equivalent to the volume of total body water in a 70-kg man, the pH of the water would fall below 3.0! But a person in normal health weathers this onslaught with only temporary and barely measurable changes in plasma pH.

Clearly, some very effective protective mechanisms must be operative to neutralize the impact of H^+ on the environment. The first line of defense is buffer systems, while the second line of defense consists of excretory mechanisms that eliminate excess H^+ or, less often, increase the concentration of H^+ when the body is threatened by alkalosis rather than acidosis.

BUFFER SYSTEMS—ONE CONTROLS ALL

The reader is probably familiar with the general principles of buffer systems, so we shall not review them here. The body has a number of such systems that cushion the effect of adding or losing H^+. These include extracellular bicarbonate/carbonic acid (HCO_3^-/H_2CO_3), phosphates and plasma proteins, intracellular hemoglobin and other proteins. In accordance with the *isohydric principle*, all of these buffer systems are in balance with each other; that is, at a given moment, each one has a ratio of undissociated acid to its anion which is in equilibrium with the pH of the environment—and the pH of the environment is the same for all the buffer systems in it. (Some modification of this statement must be made for the intracellular buffers. Just as intracellular electrolyte composition varies from that in the extracellular space—a difference that is maintained by active transport across the cell membranes—there is evidence that intracellular pH is lower than extracellular pH.)

Since all buffer systems are in balance with each other, a change in one system changes all the others. Thus the ability to regulate the ratio of one buffer combination confers control of all the other buffers and of the ambient pH.

We shall deal here with the HCO_3^-/CO_2 system, which is the vehicle through which the internal pH is controlled. The relationship between the components of this buffer and the pH can be expressed by a form of the familiar Henderson-Hasselbalch equation:

$$pH = 6.1 + \log\frac{[HCO_3^-]}{[CO_2]} \tag{1}$$

At the normal plasma pH of 7.4, the ratio of $[HCO_3^-]/[CO_2]$ (both expressed in mmol/liter) must be 20/1 in order to satisfy the equation. Since CO_2 in the plasma is often described in terms of its partial gas pressure, Pco_2, equation (1) may also be written:

$$pH = 6.1 + \log\frac{[HCO_3^-]}{0.03 \times Pco_2} \tag{2}$$

The factor 0.03 simply converts Pco_2 (expressed as mm Hg) to mmol/liter of CO_2.

Strictly speaking, $[H_2CO_3]$ should really be in the denominator of equation (1), rather than $[CO_2]$, since CO_2 is not an acid until it is hydrated to H_2CO_3:

$$CO_2 + H_2O \leftrightarrows H_2CO_3 \leftrightarrows H^+ + HCO_3^- \tag{3}$$

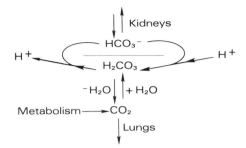

Figure 7-1. Interactions in the HCO_3^-/ CO_2 buffer system, showing the influences of kidneys and lungs.

But because CO_2 (or P_{CO_2}) is more easily measured than H_2CO_3, it has become standard practice to write equations (1) and (2) as we have shown them. The constant 6.1 used in these equations takes into account the fact that less than 1% of the CO_2 dissolved in plasma is actually hydrated to H_2CO_3.

The HCO_3^-/CO_2 combination has certain properties that make it different from other buffers and especially flexible. In most buffer systems molecules move from the numerator of the equation to the denominator and back again with the addition or subtraction of H^+, but the total number of molecules in the system does not change. In the HCO_3^-/CO_2 combination, however, new molecules can be introduced or taken away quickly and in large numbers. The kidneys can add or remove HCO_3^-, while the lungs regulate the amount of CO_2. Just as with other buffer systems, of course, numerator-to-denominator shifts (or vice versa) can take place if H^+ is added or removed. These interactions are shown diagrammatically in Figure 7-1.

Since pH is determined by the *ratio* of $[HCO_3^-]$ to $[CO_2]$, a system in which the numerator is controlled by the kidneys and the denominator by the lungs might appear to be a formula for chaos. So long as each organ is able to keep the molecular species for which it is responsible at a precise level, there is no problem, of course. But what happens when either the lungs or the kidneys are unable to keep the $[CO_2]$ or the $[HCO_3^-]$ normal? In that situation, as we shall see, each organ is able to compensate (to at least some extent) for the deficiencies of the other.

As this book concerns the kidneys, we shall focus here on their role in acid-base regulation, though it is impossible to discuss the subject adequately without some reference to the contribution of the lungs.

DEALING WITH CHALLENGES TO HOMEOSTASIS

The threat to acid-base homeostasis usually comes from the addition of acid to the body, rather than from the addition of alkali. The major source of acid is CO_2 produced by oxidation of carbon-containing compounds. This metabolic CO_2 could quickly cause a severe acidosis, but under normal circumstances the lungs act efficiently and continuously to eliminate it. In quantitative terms, the lungs are clearly number one in acid excretion.

There are, however, some acid-base problems the lungs cannot handle. Some foods, especially proteins, include phosphorus- and sulfur-containing compounds that are metabolized, in effect, to phosphoric acid and sulfuric acid. Let's follow what happens when a molecule of sulfuric acid (H_2SO_4) enters the body.

Sulfuric acid, like phosphoric acid, is too strong an acid to be tolerated in the body, so it is buffered immediately:

$$H_2SO_4 + 2NaHCO_2 \rightarrow Na_2SO_4 + 2H_2CO_3 \qquad (4)$$

$$2H_2CO_3 \rightarrow 2CO_2 + 2H_2O$$

A nasty invader has been converted to benign sodium sulfate (actually sodium and sulfate ions) and carbonic acid; the latter is largely transformed into water and CO_2, which can be eliminated by the lungs.

So the problem appears to be solved—but it really isn't. The threat of acidosis has been averted by buffering and by elimination of CO_2, but in the process two molecules of HCO_3^- have been sacrificed and not replaced. Continued loss of bicarbonate ion will result in acidosis; a glance back at the Henderson-Hasselbalch equation will show this to be true.

It might at first appear simple to replace HCO_3^-. After all, there's plenty of CO_2 around which can be converted to HCO_3^- [see equation (3)]. But the production of bicarbonate from carbon dioxide via H_2CO_3 also yields free H^+. When we consider that the concentration of HCO_3^- at the pH of the body is orders of magnitude greater than the concentration of H^+, it becomes apparent that the addition of H^+ and HCO_3^- ions in equal numbers causes a much greater relative increase in $[H^+]$ than in $[HCO_3^-]$, thus increasing acidosis rather than decreasing it. To look at the problem a bit differently, the dissociation of H_2CO_3 to H^+ and HCO_3^- would simply reverse equation (4) and return things to the threatening state of affairs that existed before sulfuric acid reacted with sodium bicarbonate.

So the replacement of HCO_3^- from ionized carbonic acid is counterproductive—*unless* the H^+ that occurs as an unwanted by-product can somehow be thrown away while the bicarbonate is retained. This is, in fact, just what the kidney does, utilizing its strategic location on a sewer line that can carry H^+ out of the body.

The Basic Process of H+ Secretion

Renal tubular cells are capable of secreting H^+ into the urinary stream along much of the length of the nephron. The effect of this process on the composition of tubular fluid is usually different in the proximal and distal parts of the nephron, but the basic mechanism of the secretion appears to be essentially

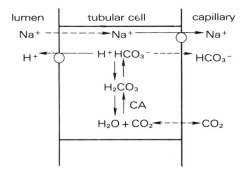

Figure 7-2. The basic process of H^+ secretion by renal tubular cells. The hydration of CO_2 to H_2CO_3 within the cells is facilitated by carbonic anhydrase (CA). Active transport across the cell membranes is shown by solid lines, passive movements by interrupted lines.

the same everywhere. Carbon dioxide, abundantly available to every cell in the body, is used as a source of H^+ and HCO_3^-, as shown in equation (3). The hydrogen ion thus produced is secreted by tubular cells into the lumen in exchange for another cation, usually sodium. The reabsorbed sodium is then transported out of the cells to the peritubular capillaries, balanced electrically by the HCO_3^- ions produced by the dissociation of H_2CO_3. These steps are shown diagrammatically in Figure 7-2. Hydration and ionization of a molecule of CO_2 thus makes possible the addition of a bicarbonate ion to the circulation, while a hydrogen ion is added to the tubular fluid.

Virtually all the H^+ entering the tubular lumen enters into one of three reactions:

1. Combination with HCO_3^-
2. Combination with buffers such as phosphate to form titratable acid
3. Combination with NH_3 to form NH_4^+

Reaction with Filtered Bicarbonate

The proximal tubular fluid contains a large quantity of filtered bicarbonate. This combines with secreted H^+ in the tubular lumen, where the reactions that took place in the tubular cell are reversed to form CO_2. The process is facilitated by carbonic anhydrase located in the brush border of the proximal tubular cells. The CO_2 produced in the lumen diffuses into the tubular cells, where it may be used as substrate to form more H^+ and HCO_3^-. So it appears that HCO_3^- is not reabsorbed from the tubular lumen as such; instead it is converted to CO_2, and the bicarbonate ions that enter the circulation are actually formed in the cells. This process is shown in Figure 7-3.

By far the greatest part of renal H^+ secretion (about 4300 mEq/day) takes place in the proximal tubules. Since H^+ has a high affinity for HCO_3^-, there can be little accumulation of free H^+ in the tubular lumen until virtually all the HCO_3^- there has been eliminated. At the end of the proximal tubule, 10 to 15% of the filtered bicarbonate still remains in the lumen under normal

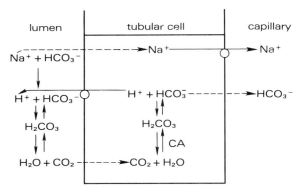

Figure 7-3. How the basic process shown in Figure 7-2 results in removal of HCO_3^- from the tubular lumen. In the proximal tubule (but not in the distal nephron) the dehydration of H_2CO_3 in the lumen to form CO_2 is catalyzed by carbonic anhydrase.

circumstances, and the pH of the tubular fluid has been reduced from 7.4 to only about 7.1.

Up to this point the H^+-secreting capacity of the renal tubules has been devoted almost entirely to the reclamation of filtered HCO_3^- to avoid the loss of bicarbonate in the urine. This is a very important function, as HCO_3^- lost in the urine has the same effect as HCO_3^- that is lost in the process of buffering strong acids.

Formation of Titratable Acid

Virtually all the filtered bicarbonate has been reclaimed by the time the tubular fluid reaches the early distal tubule. With bicarbonate out of the way, secretion of H^+ by the distal tubule can cause a substantial reduction in the pH of the tubular fluid. As the concentration of free hydrogen ions increases, H^+ associates with other buffer anions in the urine, the most important of which is HPO_4^{2-} (Fig. 7-4). The pK for this reaction is 6.8. That is,

$$pH = 6.8 + \log \frac{HPO_4^{2-}}{H_2PO_4^-}$$

At a normal serum pH of 7.4, 80% of the phosphate in glomerular filtrate is present as HPO_4^{2-} and only 20% as $H_2PO_4^-$. But when the pH of tubular fluid is lowered to 5.4, about 96% of the phosphate is present in the form of $H_2PO_4^-$. So each 100 mmol of phosphate in the tubular fluid can buffer about 76 mmol of H^+ when the pH is reduced from 7.4 to 5.4. A lesser degree of buffering may be provided by other substances in the tubular fluid, such as creatinine.

Final acidification of the urine takes place in the collecting duct, where the pH may go as low as 4.4 under some circumstances. At that point the gradient

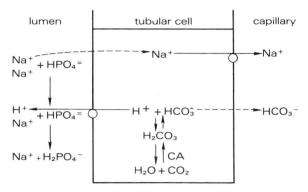

Figure 7-4. Buffering of secreted H^+ by HPO_4^{2-} in the tubular lumen.

of H^+ between tubular fluid and plasma (about 1000 to 1) appears to prevent further concentration of H^+. Considering this limitation, the buffers in tubular fluid serve an important function: By combining with H^+, they make it possible for the tubules to secrete considerable H^+ (and restore more HCO_3^- to the blood) before the lowest attainable pH is reached. Without buffers and NH_3 (to be considered next) very little H^+ secretion could take place before the minimum possible pH was reached, and the urine at a pH of 4.4 would contain only 0.04 mM of H^+ per liter. Imagine how much urine would be needed in that case to eliminate 70 mEq of H^+ daily.

The amount of H^+ present in buffered form in the urine depends upon the pH of the urine and the quantity and quality of the buffer substances it contains. Creatinine, for instance, is a less than ideal buffer because its low pK of 4.97 limits the amount of H^+ it can bind in the pH range of urine. The quantity of buffered hydrogen ion present can be determined by adding sodium hydroxide solution to a measured sample of urine until the pH has risen to 7.4. This titration simply reverses the buffering process that took place in the tubules when H^+ was secreted. The milliequivalents of hydroxide needed to restore urine pH to 7.4 are equal to those of H^+ that were added to urinary buffers. The total milliequivalents of buffered H^+ in the entire urine specimen can then be calculated. This figure, which is known as *titratable acidity*, reflects the combined contribution of all urinary buffers except NH_3. Though NH_3 acts as a buffer, it merits separate consideration for the reasons given in the following section.

Ammonium Excretion

The excretion of ammonium (NH_4^+) provides another important vehicle for the elimination of H^+; like the excretion of titratable acid, it depends heavily upon the ability of the cells in the distal nephron to reduce the pH of tubular fluid well below that of plasma.

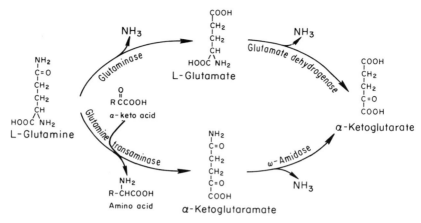

Figure 7-5. The major metabolic pathways for NH_3 formation in the renal cortex. (Reproduced by permission from D. P. Simpson, *Medicine* 50: 511, 1971.)

Some renal tubular cells have the ability to produce ammonia (NH_3). They do this primarily by deamidation of glutamine to glutamate; additional quantities of NH_3 may be liberated at times by the deamination of glutamate to α-ketoglutaric acid and by other reactions (Fig. 7-5). The arterial blood flow also brings a significant amount of ammonia to the kidneys (mostly in the form of NH_4^+).

Ammonia associates reversibly with H^+ to form ammonium:

$$NH_3 + H^+ \rightleftarrows NH_4^+$$

Since NH_3 is strongly basic, that is, an avid hydrogen-ion acceptor, this reaction goes to the right at the pH that prevails in body tissues. In blood, for instance, the concentration of NH_4^+ is approximately 100 times that of NH_3. At any pH, however, there is an equilibrium between NH_3 and NH_4^+, which is described approximately by the equation:

$$pH = 9.3 + \log \frac{[NH_3]}{[NH_4^+]}$$

Despite its low concentration, un-ionized NH_3 is very important because its lipid-solubility enables it to diffuse readily across cell membranes. Though it is produced in the cells of the proximal tubules, NH_3 passes readily into the blood, the tubular fluid, and cells of the distal tubules and collecting ducts; its concentration in all these areas is probably about the same. Within each cell or fluid space, however, the relative concentrations of NH_3 and NH_4^+ are determined by the local pH.

Figure 7-6 illustrates the theoretical distribution of NH_3 and NH_4^+ between

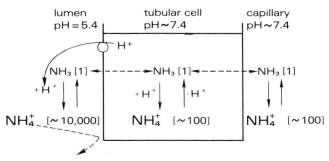

Figure 7-6. Theoretical distribution of NH_3 and NH_4^+ between a cell in the late distal tubule or collecting duct, the tubular lumen, and the peritubular capillary. Secretion of H^+ into the tubular lumen by the process shown in Figure 7-2 decreases the luminal pH. The figures in brackets show the approximate relative concentrations of NH_3 and NH_4^+ to be expected if the cell membranes are completely permeable to NH_3 and totally impermeable to NH_4^+.

a distal tubular cell and the tubular fluid. We have assumed that the pH is 7.4 within the cell and 5.4 in the tubular lumen.

Ammonia produced in the proximal tubules diffuses so freely that its concentration in the cells and in the tubular fluid is equal; this concentration is represented as [1]. Wherever it goes, most of the NH_3 will be converted to NH_4^+. Within the cell, there will be nearly 100 NH_4^+ ions for each NH_3 molecule. But within the tubular lumen this ratio will be nearly 10,000 to one because of the lower pH there. This means that the concentration of NH_4^+ in the tubular lumen is 100 times that in the cell, and not much of it can leak back into the cell because water-soluble NH_4^+ diffuses poorly across lipid cell membranes. Thus a significant amount of the NH_3/NH_4^+ available to the kidney can be trapped as NH_4^+ in acid urine. This process is referred to as *nonionic diffusion*.

Ammonia also diffuses into the renal venous blood. Because renal venous blood has a pH close to that of plasma, its concentration of NH_4^+ will be much less than that of acid urine, but its flow rate is far greater than that of urine; so venous blood carries off much of the NH_3/NH_4^+ in the renal pool. The division of NH_3/NH_4^+ between urine and venous blood is variable, depending largely on the pH of the urine (Fig. 7-7).

When NH_3 enters the tubular fluid, it combines with H^+ and, like other buffers, reduces the concentration of free hydrogen ion. The resulting decrease of the H^+ gradient between cells and tubular fluid enables the cells to secrete more H^+. Thus NH_3 diffusion facilitates the elimination of H^+ just as phosphate and the other buffer anions do. But NH_4^+ has essentially no influence on the measurement of titratable acid. This is because about 99% of total NH_3/NH_4^+ is still in its acid form—NH_4^+—when the urine is titrated back to pH 7.4. The ammonium in urine must be measured by a different method.

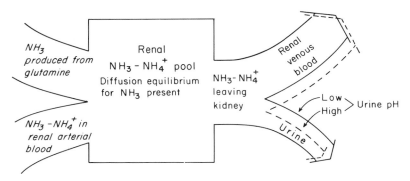

Figure 7-7. Where the NH_3/NH_4^+ in the kidney comes from and where it goes. The distribution of NH_3/NH_4^+ between renal venous blood and urine is influenced by the pH of the urine. (From D. P. Simpson, *Medicine* 50: 511, 1971.)

Total Acid Excretion

As we have already pointed out, the urinary excretion of hydrogen ion as *free* H^+ is negligible. To find out how much acid the kidneys are really excreting, we must measure both the titratable acidity (TA) of the urine and its ammonium content:

$$\text{Acid excretion} = TA + NH_4^+$$

Since there is virtually no bicarbonate in an acid urine, HCO_3^- excretion can be ignored if the pH of the urine is below 6.0. If urine is neutral or alkaline, however, it will contain a substantial amount of bicarbonate. The loss into the urine of HCO_3^- has an effect opposite to that of H^+ secretion (which increases the body's store of HCO_3^-). So in situations where there is HCO_3^- in the urine, the preceding equation needs to be modified:

$$\text{Net acid excretion} = TA + NH_4^+ - HCO_3^- \tag{5}$$

We now have an expression that applies to urine of any pH.

The net acid excretion depends upon the dietary intake of acid-forming substances. With a usual American diet, a normal adult might excrete about 70 mEq per day of H^+, of which about 30 mEq might be in the form of titratable acid and 40 mEq in the form of NH_4^+.

Meeting the Acid Test

Changing circumstances may burden the internal environment with unusual amounts of H^+. Such a challenge might come, for instance, from the consumption of a diet high in protein or other acid-forming substances. The most formidable threats to homeostasis often come from metabolic disturbances such as uncontrolled diabetes mellitus, which can liberate large quantities of strong organic acids in the body. Depletion of vital buffer systems and serious acidosis will result unless the kidneys can increase their secretion of H^+ to balance the acid entering the system.

The kidneys can respond rapidly to an acid load by secreting more H^+ and thus lowering urinary pH. (It is presumed that urine of submaximal acidity was being produced previously, as is often the case in normal subjects.) This decrease of urinary pH will cause more H^+ to be bound to urinary buffers and thus will increase the excretion of titratable acid. There will also be some increase in urinary ammonium, since the more acid urine will trap more NH_3 as NH_4^+ by the process of nonionic diffusion. These adjustments by themselves may be sufficient to neutralize the effect of an acid challenge that is small and transient.

Another weapon can be mobilized if the acid load is large and sustained: Under such circumstances the kidneys can increase their production of NH_3. The total amount of NH_4^+ in the urine really depends on two factors: the total amount of NH_3/NH_4^+ available and how it is distributed between the tubular fluid and the venous blood. Lowering the pH in the tubular fluid increases the proportion of NH_3/NH_4^+ that goes into the urine, but the total supply is quite limited. Under the stimulus of acidosis, however, the tubular cells can increase the amount of available NH_3/NH_4^+ many times.

Figure 7-8 shows the results of an experiment in which a normal subject took 240 mEq of H^+ each day for two weeks in addition to a daily diet of fixed composition. The acid load was given as ammonium chloride (NH_4Cl) because hydrochloric acid is too caustic to take by mouth, but the metabolic effect is the same, since the liver converts NH_4Cl into the equivalent of HCl and NH_3. (The NH_3 appears to be largely incorporated by the liver into urea and amino acid and thus is unrelated to production of NH_3 in the kidney.) As the figure shows, ingestion of ammonium chloride produced a prompt fall in urine pH, which was accompanied by a simultaneous increase in urinary excretion of titratable acid and ammonium. These initial responses were not sufficient to balance the effect of the continuing acid load, and the subject's bicarbonate continued to fall for several days. Meanwhile, there was a progressive increase in the daily excretion of NH_4^+. Since the urine pH hit bottom on the second day of acid loading, any increase of NH_4^+ excretion after that must have reflected an increase in the amount of NH_3/NH_4^+ available and not simply a redistribution of the preexisting supply. The increased ammonium excretion was sufficient to halt the progression of acidosis after four days, at which time the serum bicarbonate stabilized and then started to rise somewhat, despite continued ingestion of NH_4Cl.

You may note, however, that the serum bicarbonate did not return to normal during the experiment, even though renal H^+ excretion ($NH_4^+ + TA$) became almost sufficient to equal the total ingested acid. Why not? Apparently acidosis is a necessary stimulus for increased renal production of NH_3. Had

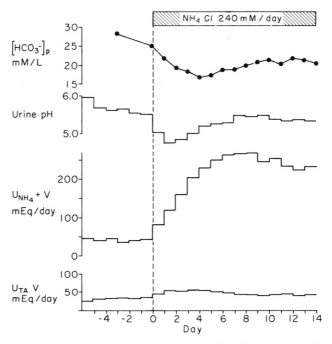

Figure 7-8. Response of a normal subject to metabolic acidosis induced by ammonium chloride, as described in the text. (From D. P. Simpson, *Medicine* 50: 516, 1971.)

the acidosis been completely corrected, NH_3 production and NH_4^+ excretion would have fallen behind the rate of acid ingestion, and the acidosis would have appeared again.

We don't know exactly how much NH_4^+ a normal human can excrete under the conditions of a severe acid stress, but the figure is probably at least 300 mEq per day (more than seven times the usual amount) and may be considerably higher. The capacity to increase the amount of NH_3 available makes the kidneys much better able to defend against acidosis than if they had to depend on the relatively fixed amounts of other buffers in the urine.

Defending Against Metabolic Alkalosis

Under most circumstances the kidneys are called upon to replace lost bicarbonate in order to avoid acidosis. Occasionally they need to deal with a surfeit of bicarbonate, which threatens the body with alkalosis. Such a situation may develop if bicarbonate-forming food or drugs are ingested in large quantities of if hydrochloric acid formed in the stomach is lost from the body by vomiting or gastric suction.

The method by which the kidneys deal with this type of alkalosis appears rather simple and highly effective under most circumstances. We have already pointed out that most of the hydrogen ion produced in renal cells is used in the proximal tubule to eliminate filtered bicarbonate from the tubular fluid and replace it in the plasma. This process takes place at a rate that will restore all the filtered bicarbonate if the plasma concentration of HCO_3^- does not exceed its normal level of about 26 mEq/liter. When plasma HCO_3^- rises above that level, the amount of HCO_3^- in glomerular filtrate increases, of course, but H^+ secretion in the proximal tubule goes on at the same rate as before. As a result, the extra bicarbonate now being filtered is abandoned in the lumen, to be lost in the urine after overwhelming the limited resorptive capacity of the distal nephron.

We can think of the proximal tubules as having a *threshold* for bicarbonate regeneration that corresponds to a normal concentration of plasma HCO_3^-. When that level is exceeded, excess bicarbonate pours over into the urine, much as water runs over a dam when its level rises above the spillway. The higher the plasma level of bicarbonate, the greater the amount that overflows into the urine. Enormous amounts of bicarbonate can be eliminated in this manner if necessary—and with no extra work by the tubular cells. The system is so effective that significant alkalosis due to HCO_3^- accumulation is virtually unknown unless the threshold for HCO_3^- resorption changes. There are some conditions in which this happens; they will be discussed shortly under the heading of Metabolic Alkalosis.

ACID-BASE DISTURBANCES IN BRIEF

As was shown in equation (1), the pH of plasma is determined by the ratio between its bicarbonate and CO_2 concentrations:

$$pH = 6.1 + \log \frac{[HCO_3^-]}{[CO_2]}$$

Thus, if plasma pH is abnormal, this ratio must be too great or too small. Such a situation can be brought about by an increase or a decrease in $[HCO_3^-]$ or $[CO_2]$ or some combination of these. If only one basic aberration is present, we are dealing with one of the so-called *primary acid-base disturbances*. Such disturbances may result from too much or too little CO_2 or from too much or too little HCO_3^-, and they are named accordingly as shown as Table 7-1. In their pure, uncorrected forms, these abnormalities are described as *uncompensated* respiratory acidosis, *uncompensated* metabolic alkalosis, and so on.

Table 7-1. Hallmarks of the Primary Acid-Base Disorders

	CO_2	HCO_3^-
Too much	Respiratory acidosis	Metabolic alkalosis
Too little	Respiratory alkalosis	Metabolic acidosis

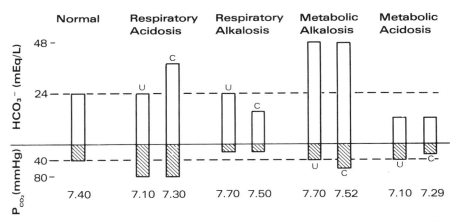

Figure 7-9. Representative values for HCO_3^- and Pco_2 in the primary acid-base distur-bances. The bars marked U show the uncompensated state which would be seen if $[HCO_3^-]$ were held constant in primary respiratory disorders and if Pco_2 remained normal in primary metabolic disturbances. Bars marked C show the compensation that usually takes place in a chronic disturbance. Figures below the bars show pH. Though the usual molar ratio of $HCO_3^-/CO_2 = 20/1$ at pH 7.4, the bars representing CO_2 have been expanded here for graphic purposes.

While the lungs govern the plasma content of CO_2 and the kidneys control the concentration of bicarbonate, their roles are not entirely independent. Like good singers in a duet, each one must be prepared to modify its part if the other cannot perform as expected. So if the lungs are unable to maintain a normal concentration of CO_2, the kidneys are likely to change the concentra-tion of HCO_3^- in the direction that will bring the pH back toward normal. The primary respiratory disturbance is then said to be *compensated*. Similarly, if the kidneys cannot maintain a normal level of bicarbonate, the lungs respond to produce a *compensated* metabolic disturbance. These compensatory adjust-ments are illustrated in Figure 7-9. Generally, they do not bring the pH all the way back to normal, though that happens at times in the primary respiratory disturbances.

We cannot deal fully with acid-base disturbances in a few pages; many books are devoted solely to this subject. However, we shall outline the primary disturbances with their common causes and the compensation that usually occurs, giving special attention to situations in which acidosis is caused by dysfunction of the kidneys themselves.

Respiratory Acidosis

Respiratory acidosis occurs in situations where there is decreased alveolar ventilation. This may happen with depression of the central nervous system and in certain pulmonary diseases. The hypoventilation results in an increase of plasma carbon dioxide concentration, which decreases the ratio of bicarbonate to carbon dioxide, lowering plasma pH. (Some of the additional carbonic acid formed will be neutralized by other buffer systems and thus converted to more HCO_3^-, but the ratio HCO_3^-/CO_2 will still be decreased because of a relatively greater rise in the denominator.)

The kidneys respond to respiratory acidosis by secreting more H^+ and thus generating additional HCO_3^-. The presence of more CO_2 in all tissues, including the tubular cells, may provide the stimulus as well as the substrate for this increased activity. The additional bicarbonate produced by the kidneys raises the ratio HCO_3^-/CO_2, compensating partially for the respiratory acidosis (Fig. 7-9). This process may take several days.

Respiratory Alkalosis

Overventilation of the pulmonary alveoli may be caused by some diseases of the central nervous system, by emotional disturbances, and by certain drugs or poisons. This causes a decrease in plasma carbon dioxide concentration, an increase in the HCO_3^-/CO_2 ratio, and therefore a rise in plasma pH. (Other buffer systems will convert some HCO_3^- to H_2CO_3, but the ratio will still be increased.)

In the kidneys, the process just described for respiratory acidosis is reversed. There is decreased secretion of H^+, and some filtered HCO_3^- is then lost in the urine. The resulting reduction of plasma HCO_3^- moves the ratio HCO_3^-/CO_2 back toward normal (Fig. 7-9).

Metabolic Alkalosis

Metabolic alkalosis, characterized by a primary increase in plasma bicarbonate concentration, may be caused by the excessive intake of alkaline-forming substances or, more commonly, by loss of gastric acid from the body in large amounts. In the stomach as in the kidney, secretion of a hydrogen ion is accompanied by the addition of a bicarbonate ion to the plasma. Under normal circumstances, gastric H^+ reacts with alkaline fluids in the intestine and does not leave the body, so the secretory activity of the stomach has no net effect on acid-base homeostasis. When acid gastric juice is removed by persistent vomiting or suction, however, the stomach becomes an H^+-secreting and an HCO_3^--generating organ of major importance. Under such circumstances, the addition of bicarbonate to the circulation tends to raise the HCO_3^-/CO_2 ratio and the plasma pH. The lungs may compensate partially by reducing alveolar ventilation, thus allowing CO_2 concentration to rise somewhat (Fig. 7-9).

As we have already mentioned, the kidneys are marvelously efficient, under ordinary circumstances, at preventing metabolic alkalosis; excess bicarbonate can be spilled into the urine in huge amounts. For this reason, it is difficult to produce a significant alkalosis in a person with normal kidneys by adminis-

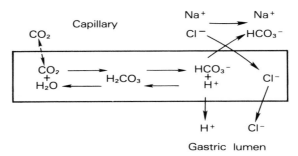

Figure 7-10. Diagram to show how secretion of HCl into the gastric lumen is accompanied by the addition of $NaHCO_3$ to the blood.

tering sodium bicarbonate. Why then does metabolic alkalosis often result from losing large amounts of gastric juice? It can happen only because certain circumstances change the renal threshold for HCO_3^- resorption.

Let's follow the sequence of events in a person with persistent vomiting, which also prevents the retention of food. Hydrochloric acid ($H^+ + Cl^-$) is lost in the vomitus; its production leaves behind HCO_3^- and the Na^+ which had been balancing the secreted Cl^- (Fig. 7-10). If the process continues, the serum HCO_3^- concentration begins to rise. As it does, filtered bicarbonate above the threshold level is allowed to escape into the urine with sodium as its usual cation, and alkalosis is averted.

So the loss of HCl from the stomach is balanced by the excretion of $NaHCO_3$ by the kidneys. Note, however, that NaCl has been lost in the process:

$$\underset{\text{(lost from stomach)}}{H^+ + Cl^-} \quad + \quad \underset{\text{(excreted by kidneys)}}{Na^+ + HCO_3^-} \rightarrow NaCl + H_2O + CO_2$$

If vomiting is prolonged, a significant depletion of $Na^+ + Cl^-$ may occur, resulting in a reduction of the extracellular fluid volume, which has important effects. One of these is increased retrieval of filtered HCO_3^- in the proximal tubule, just as many filtered substances are reabsorbed to a greater extent when there is extracellular volume depletion. In effect, the threshold for bicarbonate excretion is raised, allowing the plasma level to climb higher before HCO_3^- is lost into the urine. Other effects of volume reduction are increased aldosterone secretion and more avid sodium resorption all along the nephron.

The kidney now has a dilemma. If HCO_3^- is excreted to correct the alkalosis, a cation, usually Na^+, must be lost also, but this will aggravate the volume depletion problem. The kidney's priorities in this situation are pretty clear: The extracellular fluid volume must be protected first, and the acid-base problem will have to wait. In effect, volume depletion prevents the kidney from correcting the alkalosis. Conversely, a significant degree of metabolic alkalosis is not likely to be established and maintained in a person with normal kidneys unless sodium depletion (or other stimulus to HCO_3^- resorption) is also present.

In addition, other important things happen in such a situation. Plasma chloride is depressed in metabolic alkalosis, and the reduced amount of chloride in glomerular filtrate is mostly gone when the tubular fluid reaches the distal nephron. Therefore, much of the remaining sodium in the fluid is balanced by poorly resorbable anions. This means that if the sodium is to be reclaimed—and it must be—another cation must be secreted in its place. The tubular cells appear to have very limited options: they can secrete H^+, K^+, or (usually) both.

Secretion of H^+ into the distal tubular fluid of a subject with metabolic alkalosis seems misguided. Indeed, it *is* inappropriate if seen only in the context of acid-base balance. Such secretion adds HCO_3^- to the plasma, where there is too much of it already. And it may cause the urine pH to be low—the so-called *paradoxical aciduria* of metabolic alkalosis. But it isn't paradoxical in terms of volume regulation, since those hydrogen ions in the urine make possible the recovery of sodium.

Secretion of K^+ into the urine may be sufficient to cause potassium depletion, a problem that often accompanies metabolic alkalosis. The deficiency of K^+ creates some difficulties of its own. In addition to systemic consequences, potassium depletion raises the threshold for bicarbonate recovery in the proximal tubule and may enhance H^+ secretion in the distal nephron as well, thus sustaining the alkalosis.

Metabolic alkalosis in a person with good renal function can usually be corrected simply by providing sodium chloride to expand the extracellular fluid space. Relieved of the obligation to recover all filtered sodium, the kidneys can then excrete the excess bicarbonate with sodium cations. In situations where a serious degree of potassium deficiency has developed, it may be necessary to replace K^+ also before alkalosis can be reversed. Some investigators believe that it is really a deficiency of chloride (produced by vomiting HCl) that prevents the kidneys from correcting metabolic alkalosis. According to their view, sodium chloride solutions are effective in treatment because of the chloride they contain—not simply because of their sodium.

Metabolic Acidosis

In patients with metabolic acidosis there is a primary decrease in the concentration of plasma bicarbonate. This may be caused by the addition to the body of large quantities of acid (other than CO_2), by impaired renal ability to excrete H^+ and regenerate HCO_3^-, or by a combination of both factors. Clinical problems characterized by metabolic acidosis include diabetic ketoacidosis, some types of poisoning or drug overdose, a major reduction in the number of functioning nephrons (renal failure) and more specific tubular dysfunctions (renal tubular acidosis).

The loss of plasma bicarbonate common to all of these situations reduces the HCO_3^-/CO_2 ratio and thus the plasma pH. The kidneys may be working hard to restore bicarbonate to its normal levels and correct the acidosis, as described earlier in this chapter, and in some cases they will eventually succeed; but the presence of decreased bicarbonate and decreased pH shows that the situation is, at least temporarily, not completely under control. Now it is the lungs that compensate. Stimulated by the fall in blood pH, a sensitive respiratory center in the brain directs an increase in alveolar ventilation, reducing the plasma CO_2 concentration. This brings the HCO_3^-/CO_2 ratio back toward normal (Fig. 7-9). Unlike renal compensation, respiratory compensation is very rapid, almost immediate.

Acidosis Caused by Renal Dysfunction

In some situations there is acidosis because the kidneys are unable to maintain normal bicarbonate levels even under ordinary conditions when only moderate acid loads need to be excreted. Acidosis due to inadequate renal performance results most commonly from a loss of functioning renal tissue, which may be caused by a variety of diseases. This type of metabolic acidosis is a part of the picture of renal failure and will be described in Chapter 12. A different kind of renal acidosis, which usually occurs in the absence of generalized kidney damage, will be described briefly here.

Renal tubular acidosis (RTA) is a term applied to disorders in which the kidneys are unable to excrete H^+ normally, even though they function adequately in most other respects. The common feature of these problems is a metabolic acidosis, typically mild or moderate, often with normal serum creatinine levels. It is now recognized that there are two distinct kinds of RTA, and a recently described disorder has been proposed as an additional type.

Distal RTA is caused by a reduced ability of the distal nephron to acidify the urine. Whereas normal kidneys can respond to acidosis by decreasing the pH of urine to 5.0 or less, as seen in Figure 7-8, persons with distal RTA are not able to produce a urine with a pH below about 6.0. It is not certain whether this reflects a failure of the collecting ducts to generate enough H^+, an inability to secrete H^+ against a large gradient, or an abnormal back-leak of H^+ from the tubular fluid.

Under normal circumstances, the amount of phosphate in the urine of an individual is fairly constant, so the titratable acidity of the urine varies with its hydrogen-ion concentration. A restricted ability to acidify the urine means that less H^+ can be excreted as titratable acid and also that less of the renal NH_3/NH_4^+ pool enters the urine. As a result, bicarbonate regeneration suffers, and metabolic acidosis develops. The acidosis stimulates the production of NH_3 by the tubular cells, allowing more hydrogen ions to be excreted as NH_4^+ at any prevailing pH of the urine; this compensates to some extent for the reduction of titratable acidity. Another effect of chronic acidosis is that a small amount of each day's H^+ production is buffered by bone tissue.

The clinical consequences of distal RTA may include abnormal loss of potassium and calcium in the urine, formation of renal stones, calcification of kidney tissue, bone disease (especially in children), and the manifestations of potassium depletion.

Distal RTA is also called *Type I RTA* because it was the first kind of renal tubular acidosis to be recognized. This disorder may be hereditary or sporadic, or it may appear in connection with other conditions such as hyperglobulinemia, hyperparathyroidism, either a deficiency or excess of vitamin D, exposure to amphotericin-B and some other drugs, and chronic hydronephrosis.

Proximal RTA results from an inability of proximal tubular cells to secrete adequate amounts of H^+. You will recall that most renal H^+ secretion takes place in the proximal tubules and accounts for the regeneration of 85 to 90% of filtered bicarbonate. When this process is defective, an excessive amount of HCO_3^- is passed downstream. Since the distal nephron has a relatively small capacity for H^+ secretion, it is unlikely to reclaim all of the HCO_3^- that is now presented to it. So bicarbonate is lost into the urine, and a metabolic acidosis ensues.

Proximal RTA has a self-limiting feature, however. As serum bicarbonate falls due to losses in the urine, filtered HCO_3^- also decreases until a level is reached where the proximal tubule is able to recover virtually all of it. When this happens, the normal cells of the distal nephron are no longer inundated by spilled-over HCO_3^-, so it becomes possible for them to acidify the urine in a normal manner. At this point the renal net acid secretion [equation (5)] may be normal and approximately equal to daily H^+ production, but only so long as serum bicarbonate remains low.

Proximal RTA may occur as an isolated defect, but more commonly it is found in association with other functional abnormalities of the proximal tubule, such as decreased resorption of glucose, amino acids, or phosphate. When several of these defects occur together, the name *Fanconi syndrome* is often used to describe the picture. Proximal RTA is a feature of a number of diseases such as myeloma, cystinosis, fructose intolerance, galactosemia, or heavy-metal toxicity. Sometimes, however, it is hereditary or has no evident cause.

Proximal RTA is also called *Type II RTA* because it was the second type of renal tubular acidosis to be described.

As the reader may have already perceived, one important difference between the two types of renal tubular acidosis just described relates to the acidity of the urine and what it means. Patients with distal RTA are unable to produce a strongly acid urine under any circumstances, while those with proximal RTA can acidify the urine well—but only if serum bicarbonate is adequately depressed. It follows that an accurate urine pH measurement of 5.2 or less excludes the diagnosis of distal RTA but not of proximal RTA.

Another important difference is that the acidosis of distal RTA can be treated effectively with relatively small amounts of alkali; only enough need be given to balance the body's H^+ production each day, thus making it unnecessary for the kidneys to excrete H^+. On the other hand, the treatment of proximal RTA requires large doses of alkali because of the decreased threshold for bicarbonate excretion; trying to raise the serum bicarbonate in such patients is like trying to fill a bucket that has a large hole in its side.

An acidosis resembling that seen in RTA is commonly associated with *hyporeninemic hypoaldosteronism*. As the name implies, this condition is characterized by low plasma levels of both renin and aldosterone. Since renin is an important stimulus for the release of aldosterone, the low levels of aldosterone are probably caused by a primary deficiency of renin. When aldosterone acts on the cells of the distal nephron to stimulate sodium resorption, secretion of K^+ and H^+ are promoted. We would then expect a lack of aldosterone to reduce the secretion of H^+, which might result in acidosis. However, it appears that the crucial factor that allows acidosis to develop in this setting may really be a failure of the tubular cells to produce enough NH_3 (for reasons that are still being sought).

Some investigators have labeled this condition *Type IV RTA.** But unlike Types I and II RTA, hyporeninemic hypoaldosteronism is often found in persons who already have destructive renal disease, such as that caused by diabetes mellitus, with impaired glomerular filtration. In such patients the generalized renal disease may have damaged the renin-secreting cells in the juxtaglomerular apparatus.

Renal Acidosis and the Anion Gap

Under normal conditions the plasma concentration of sodium (about 140 mEq/liter) exceeds the combined concentrations of chloride (about 102 mEq/liter) and bicarbonate (about 26 mEq/liter) by about 12 mEq/liter. This difference is referred to as the *anion gap* (AG), and it becomes even larger if lesser cations like potassium, calcium, and magnesium are added to the sodium. In reality, there cannot be more milliequivalents of cations than of anions, so the term *anion gap* is really a misnomer. The necessary negative charges are provided by plasma proteins, phosphate, sulfate, organic acids, and other anions that are not usually measured. So the anion gap, as the term is usually used, refers only to the difference between sodium and the *measured* anions Cl^- and HCO_3^-:

$$AG = [Na^+] - [Cl^-] - [HCO_3^-]$$

The hallmark of metabolic acidosis is a decrease of plasma bicarbonate. Since metabolic acidosis by itself does not change the plasma sodium concentration, electrical balance must be preserved by an increase in the concentra-

---

*What happened to Type III RTA? It appeared in the medical literature some years ago, but the name was largely abandoned when it was recognized that the condition it described was really a variant of distal RTA.

tion of some other anion to compensate for the decrease of [HCO_3^-]. Sometimes this is accomplished by an increase in [Cl^-]. In that case the sum of [Cl^-] and [HCO_3^-] remains at its usual level, and the gap between these anions and [Na^+] does not change. In many cases, however, the HCO_3^- is replaced by an anion that is not usually measured. This results in an increased anion gap.

The presence or absence of an elevated anion gap in a patient with metabolic acidosis can be a valuable clue to the cause of the acidosis. This is best shown by a few examples:

1. In uncontrolled diabetes mellitus there is overproduction of acetoacetic acid and β-hydroxybutyric acid. The H^+ from these strong organic acids is buffered by plasma HCO_3^-. The result is that plasma [HCO_3^-] falls, while the usually unmeasured anions acetoacetate and β-hydroxybutyrate accumulate in plasma faster than they can be metabolized or excreted. Since [Cl^-] is not affected, an increased anion gap develops.

2. Renal failure is typically characterized by impairment of both glomerular and tubular functions and by metabolic acidosis. Metabolism of proteins in the body liberates sulfuric and phosphoric acids. Continued production of these acids causes serum bicarbonate to fall because the tubules collectively have a decreased capacity to excrete H^+ and regenerate HCO_3^-. At the same time, plasma concentrations of sulfate and phosphate usually rise because of decreased glomerular filtration. So the loss of HCO_3^- is accompanied by an increase of unmeasured anions, and the anion gap increases.

In both of the preceding examples it must be emphasized that the acid anions in the plasma—acetoacetate, β-hydroxybutyrate, sulfate, or phosphate—are not causing acidosis. The hydrogen ions that came with them did the damage, and the residual anions are like the spent cartridges found after a gun fight. But just as an expert can use empty cartridges to tell what kind of bullets were fired, we can often gain information about the cause of an acidosis by identifying the anions that have replaced bicarbonate. In example 1, for instance, the discovery of increased amounts of acetoacetate or β-hydroxybutyrate in the plasma would make it highly likely that the patient had diabetic ketoacidosis.

3. Severe diarrhea can cause metabolic acidosis due to the loss of bicarbonate in the stool. There are no unmeasured anions being added to the plasma in this situation; instead, the concentration of Cl^- rises as that of HCO_3^- falls, and no anion gap develops.

4. In renal tubular acidosis of any type, serum bicarbonate falls below normal because HCO_3^- is being lost in the urine or not being regenerated adequately by the tubules. If glomerular function is normal, there is no accumulation of unmeasured anions. As in the preceding example, [Cl^-] rises as [HCO_3^-] decreases, and there is no anion gap. Patients with chronic renal failure may also have acidosis without an anion gap at some stage of

their disease. This occurs if the damaged tubules can no longer regenerate HCO_3^- well enough to maintain a normal plasma bicarbonate level while glomerular function remains adequate to prevent the accumulation of unmeasured anions such as sulfate.

Thus the lack of an increased anion gap can help to distinguish renal tubular acidosis and a few other conditions from the more common causes of metabolic acidosis.

BIBLIOGRAPHY

R. G. Narins and M. Emmett. Simple and mixed acid-base disorders: A practical approach. *Medicine* 59: 161–187, 1980.

F. C. Rector, Jr., and M. G. Cogan. The renal acidoses. *Hosp. Prac.* 15: 99–111, April 1980.

D. P. Simpson. Control of hydrogen ion homeostasis and renal acidosis. *Medicine* 50: 503–541, 1971.

A more detailed discussion of the principles of buffer systems and their role in the body may be found in a number of texts, such as the following:

R. F. Pitts. *Physiology of the kidney and body fluids,* 3rd ed. Chicago: Year Book Medical Publishers, 1974.

B. D. Rose. *Clinical physiology of acid-base and electrolyte disorders.* New York: McGraw-Hill, 1977.

H. Valtin. *Renal function: Mechanisms preserving fluid and solute balance in health.* Boston: Little, Brown, 1973.

8

How the Kidneys Regulate Potassium Excretion

The human diet contains a large and variable amount of potassium (K^+), estimated to be about 60 mEq/day for the average American. So far as we know, virtually all of this potassium is absorbed indiscriminately from the gastrointestinal tract whether the body needs it or not. It falls to the kidneys, therefore, to excrete enough K^+ each day so that the potassium we eat and absorb will not accumulate and poison us. At the same time, the kidneys must retain the right amount of K^+ to permit proper operation of the vital functions that depend on it.

In some respects the regulation of potassium balance is more complex than that of sodium. Sodium is confined almost exclusively to the extracellular fluid, and the kidneys need only regulate its excretion to maintain suitable conditions for life in that compartment. In the case of potassium, however, the amount in the extracellular fluid comprises only about 2% of the total amount in the body, the other 98% being found in the cells. It is not enough for the kidneys to respond only to the potassium level in the extracellular fluid, since this concentration is not always an accurate reflection of the much larger total body stores of potassium.

Other things being equal, it is true that a significant excess of total body potassium is likely to be accompanied by an increase of plasma K^+, and a major deficit of total body potassium will usually cause plasma K^+ to fall. Yet there are situations in which the usual intercompartmental distribution of potassium is altered, making the plasma K^+ concentration an unreliable indicator. In some types of metabolic acidosis, for instance, intracellular K^+ enters the extracellular fluid—perhaps in exchange for hydrogen ions that move into the cells to be buffered—and raises the plasma K^+ concentration even though total body potassium stores may be normal or low. A shift of K^+ ions in the opposite direction may occur in alkalosis. Some hormones, notably aldosterone and insulin, may also alter the distribution of potassium. So in order to control potassium appropriately the kidneys must be responsive to intracellular as well as extracellular K^+.

113

The requirements for potassium regulation are exacting. The potassium concentration within cells must be maintained at its normal high level, about 150 mEq/liter of cell water. The extracellular potassium concentration must be kept within a narrow range, normally about 3.5 to 5.5 mEq/liter. The consequences of significant departures from these norms are potentially disastrous, because neuromuscular conduction throughout the body—depolarization and repolarization of nerves and muscles—depends on the relationship between intracellular and extracellular potassium concentration. For instance, an extracellular potassium concentration that is either too high or too low can cause profound weakness or paralysis. Even more alarming are the cardiac consequences of hypo- or hyperkalemia: changes in cardiac conduction, demonstrable by electrocardiography, which may evolve with little warning into fatal arrhythmias. It is no exaggeration to say that controlling the amount and distribution of potassium in the body is a matter of life and death.

Although this chapter will focus on the role of the kidneys, we cannot really understand potassium regulation unless we also keep in mind the factors causing it to enter or leave the cell—especially since the distribution of potassium in the body influences its excretion by the kidneys.

HOW DO THE KIDNEYS DEAL WITH POTASSIUM?

Considering the explosion of information in the past two decades and the amount of research still taking place, no author in his right mind would presume to offer "the last word" about the renal excretion of potassium. Though we will suggest some unifying concepts that may help to make some sense out of the subject, the reader should be aware that the renal handling of potassium is incompletely understood and in some respects controversial. Sophisticated micropuncture techniques have yielded much information, but some of these findings only make it evident that renal K^+ transport is more complicated than once thought. For instance, it is now apparent that the distal tubule, a critical site for potassium regulation, is not a uniform structure and probably does not function in the same way throughout its entire length. Structural and functional differences between the distal tubules of various species make it unlikely that information obtained from rats and dogs will give a precise picture of events in the human kidney. And even within the same species we cannot be sure that superficial nephrons, whose proximal and distal tubules are accessible to micropuncture, are treating potassium in the same way as the juxtamedullary nephrons, which can be sampled only where their loops of Henle turn at the tip of the renal papilla.

Despite these complexities, some things can be said with confidence about the fate of K^+ within the nephron. Since the potassium ion is small and bound very little if at all to plasma proteins, its concentration in glomerular filtrate is close to that in plasma. The total amount of potassium filtered does not approach the enormous quantities of sodium delivered to the tubules simply

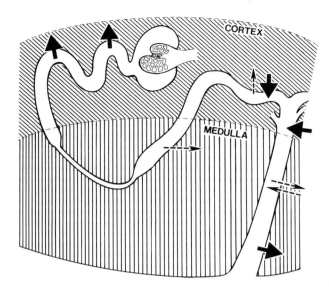

Figure 8-1. Locations of potassium resorption and secretion in a superficial (cortical) nephron and a collecting duct, shown very schematically here. Solid arrows show generally accepted sites and directions of potassium transport. Dotted arrows show probable sites and directions of potassium movement. (Redrawn and modified from F. Wright and G. Giebisch, *Am. J. Physiol.* 235: F517, 1978.)

because the plasma concentration of K^+ is so much less than that of sodium. Even so, the daily filtration of potassium under normal conditions is ten times the amount that needs to be excreted to maintain homeostasis on an average diet. Only a small fraction of this filtered K^+ appears in the urine, and almost none at all under circumstances of potassium deprivation, so we know that the tubules can reabsorb potassium efficiently.

It is also clear that the renal tubules can secrete K^+. Perhaps the most convincing evidence of this was the demonstration that under some circumstances the quantity of potassium in the urine is substantially in excess of the amount that could have been filtered. This phenomenon may be seen when there is a drastic reduction in glomerular filtration rate together with a liberal potassium intake. Such conditions may seem esoteric, but we know now from micropuncture studies that secretion of K^+ by the tubules also plays an important part in the normal day-to-day regulation of potassium excretion.

Figure 8-1 summarizes present thinking about the general sites of potassium resorption and secretion in a superficial nephron. (We don't really know whether juxtamedullary nephrons function in a similar way.) It appears that potassium resorption takes place in most parts of the nephron and that both passive and active mechanisms contribute to this process. In the proximal tubule, for instance, the removal of large quantities of tubular fluid (in response to the resorption of sodium and chloride) would tend to raise the

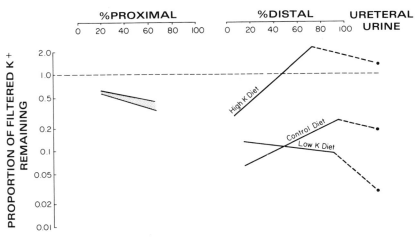

Figure 8-2. Changes in the potassium content of tubular fluid in the rat, showing the influence of dietary K^+ on the removal or addition of K^+ by different parts of the nephron. Micropuncture was used to study rats that had been maintained on a control diet, a low-K^+ diet, or a high-K^+ diet. The sites sampled are represented on the horizontal scale as a percentage of the distance along the proximal or distal tubule. Tubular-fluid potassium, on the vertical scale, is shown as the proportion of filtered K^+ remaining. A downward-sloping line indicates net resorption of K^+, while an upward slope reflects net secretion. Potassium resorption in the proximal tubule was similar for all dietary groups, as shown by the shaded area. Potassium secretion in the animals on the high-K^+ diet was facilitated in this experiment by the infusion of potassium chloride, sodium sulfate and a carbonic-anhydrase inhibitor during the collection periods. (This graph is a composite redrawn from the work of G. Malnic, R. M. Klose, and G. Giebisch in *Am. J. Physiol.* 206: 674–686, 1964.)

concentration of potassium left behind in the lumen, creating a chemical gradient that would drive potassium out of the tubular fluid. On the other hand, there is evidence that in some situations the potassium concentration within the proximal tubule is too low to have been achieved by passive diffusion alone and that active resorption (against an electrochemical gradient) must have taken place. Whatever the mechanism, only about 10% of the filtered K^+ is still present in the earliest part of the distal tubule that can be sampled by micropuncture.

In the distal tubule and collecting duct potassium may be removed from or added to the tubular fluid. Unlike the resorption in the earlier parts of the nephron, which does not seem to be influenced by the body's need to excrete or to conserve potassium, the processes in the distal tubule are quite responsive to the overall state of potassium balance. Figure 8-2, based on micropuncture studies of rats, shows how the potassium content of fluid in the distal tubules varies with the amount of potassium in the diet. The distal tubule and the cortical collecting duct now appear to be the places in the

nephron where the major regulation of renal K⁺ excretion takes place. Let's
take a closer look at the distal tubule.

SECRETION MAKES THE DIFFERENCE

We can see from Figure 8-2 that the options available to the distal tubule
range from a small net additional resorption of potassium to a massive
secretion that may approach or even exceed the amount of potassium reabsorbed more proximally. Surprising though it may seem, this secretory
mechanism—an essential step in a critical regulatory process—appears to be
passive rather than active. That is, the movement of potassium into tubular
fluid is not accomplished by an ion pump for potassium; instead it is a
response to electrical forces and a chemical gradient. But as we shall see, some
of these electrical and chemical forces are determined by the body's state of
potassium balance.

Figure 8-3 represents a cell from the distal tubule in relation to the tubular
lumen and the peritubular fluid. It is important to remember that renal
tubular cells share many of the characteristics of cells elsewhere. In particular,
their internal potassium concentration is quite high and sodium concentration
very low. These chemical features are maintained by the constant action of
energy-requiring ion pumps located on the peritubular side of the cell. You

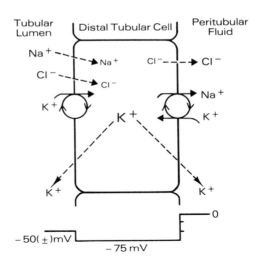

Figure 8-3. Representation of a cell near the end of the distal tubule of a rat, showing
movements of K⁺, Na⁺, and Cl⁻. Solid arrows represent active transport; dashed
arrows show passive movements. The electrical potential of the cell interior and the
tubular lumen in millivolts (mV) are shown in relation to the peritubular fluid, which is
assumed to have a potential of zero. The amount of negative potential in the tubular
lumen may vary considerably depending on experimental conditions.

should also note that the tubular lumen is electrically negative in relation to the peritubular fluid and that the interior of the cell is even more negative.

Ultimately only two forces appear to determine how much potassium is secreted passively by the distal tubular cells into the tubular lumen:

1. The relative concentrations of potassium in the cells and in the lumen. Because of the high levels of potassium within the cells, the concentration gradient favors its movement from the cells into the lumen. The *amount* of difference between cells and lumen, and therefore the chemical force favoring secretion, can vary depending on circumstances, however.
2. The electrical potential in the tubular lumen relative to that in the cells. Since the cell is negative in relation to the lumen and the potassium ion has a positive charge, the electrical force favors resorption of potassium from the lumen. Like the potassium gradient, the electrical difference between lumen and cells can change with conditions.

For practical purposes the amount of potassium secreted or absorbed in the distal tubule appears to depend on the balance of these two factors.

Strict accuracy requires that we hedge this statement with some minor reservations: There is some evidence for an active resorptive potassium pump in the distal tubule, as shown in Figure 8-3. Its influence appears minor compared with that of potassium secretion. And some evidence suggests that the permeability of the luminal membrane may change in response to aldosterone. Such a change, if it really happens, would influence the rate of potassium transfer but not its direction.

Conditions known to promote potassium secretion are shown in Table 8-1. We have arranged them according to the physiological mechanisms through which they may exert their effects, though some of these explanations are

Table 8-1. Factors Promoting Renal K^+ Secretion

I. Increased concentration gradient of K^+ (from tubular cells to lumen)
   A. Increased intracellular K^+
      1. Increased total-body K^+
      2. Alkalosis (?)
      3. Increased aldosterone
   B. Accelerated removal of K^+ from lumen
      1. Increased flow of fluid in distal tubule

II. Increased electronegativity of distal tubular lumen
   A. Increased avidity of distal sodium reabsorption
      1. Increased aldosterone
   B. More sodium available for distal reabsorption (?)
   C. Poorly absorbed anions in lumen

III. Increased permeability of luminal membrane in distal tubule (?)
   A. Increased aldosterone (?)

based more on speculation than on sound evidence. For instance, although K^+ may enter cells during alkalosis, it has not been proved that intracellular K^+ is increased to any important degree or that this is responsible for increasing renal potassium excretion. Some of the other conditions listed in Table 8-1 also deserve further explanation.

Aldosterone is an extremely important factor in potassium secretion, which it may influence through several mechanisms. The best established of these is its ability to stimulate sodium resorption in the distal tubule (see Chapter 5). It was once believed that there is an equal exchange in the distal tubule: one potassium ion secreted for each sodium ion reabsorbed. We know now that this is not so and that the amount of sodium reabsorbed is much greater than the amount of potassium secreted. Nevertheless, these two processes are related—probably because the resorption of positively charged sodium ions leaves the lumen relatively more negative, thus promoting potassium secretion. It appears that aldosterone may also increase intracellular K^+ concentration by stimulating the ion pumps in peritubular cell membranes.

Conditions in which unusually large amounts of fluid are delivered to the distal tubule are often accompanied by large urinary potassium losses, and it has been shown by micropuncture studies that distal K^+ secretion is flow-related under some circumstances. Presumably a high rate of flow through the distal tubule carries away secreted potassium quickly and prevents a high luminal concentration from developing.

A high rate of flow in the distal tubule may occur during an osmotic diuresis and in any other circumstances where there is decreased proximal resorption. Under such conditions, there is increased delivery of both sodium and fluid to the distal tubule. The volume of fluid appears to be important, but it is possible that the increased amount of sodium available for resorption in the lumen of the distal tubule may also influence K^+ secretion. The relationship between sodium resorption and potassium secretion in the distal tubule has already been discussed, and it seems to be real. The question is whether additional sodium beyond the amount normally present will lead to further K^+ secretion. In real life it is difficult to separate this possible effect from that of increased tubular fluid flow alone.

It should be mentioned that the opposite change—inadequate delivery of sodium to the distal nephron—can have startling and clinically important effects on potassium secretion. In situations where extracellular fluid volume is depleted and the kidneys are underperfused, the proportion of sodium and tubular fluid reabsorbed in the proximal nephron appears to be increased, leaving relatively little to be delivered distally. Under such circumstances there may be a failure of K^+ secretion and dangerous hyperkalemia, despite high levels of aldosterone. Correction of the underperfusion remedies the problem. Here again, we cannot be sure whether to blame poor delivery of sodium to the distal tubule or a decreased flow of tubular fluid, since they occur together.

The anions that reach the distal tubule with sodium can have an important influence on the secretion of potassium and hydrogen ions. Resorption of a sodium cation must be balanced electrically by resorption of an anion or the secretion of a cation—K^+ or H^+ in this case. Whether an anion leaves the lumen or a cation enters it may be determined by the ease with which the anions in the tubular fluid can be reabsorbed with sodium. Because cell walls are relatively permeable to chloride, a large preponderance of this anion reduces distal secretion of K^+ and H^+ when sodium is reabsorbed, since most sodium cations will be accompanied by chloride anions. Anions to which the distal tubule is less permeable, such as sulfate or the antibiotic carbenicillin, tend to lag behind as sodium is reabsorbed. Their wayward presence, together with the resorption of sodium, increases the electrical negativity of the tubular lumen and enhances secretion of K^+ and H^+ cations. This phenomenon is likely to occur whenever another anion replaces tubular-fluid chloride in significant amounts, since most anions are poorly absorbed in comparison with chloride.

Table 8-1 and this discussion have emphasized the factors that promote renal potassium secretion. The absence of these factors or opposite influences (such as a decrease of total body potassium) will usually reduce distal K^+ secretion. An exception is acidosis, which like alkalosis may stimulate urinary K^+ excretion.

PHYSIOLOGY AT THE BEDSIDE

With this background in mind, it is easy to see how some clinical events influence the urinary excretion of potassium. As an example, let's consider the well-known potassium-losing effect of potent diuretics such as the thiazides. Remember first that diuretics are often used in people whose kidneys are not excreting enough sodium; the mechanisms for sodium resorption in such patients are likely to be working overtime, including stimulation of the distal tubules by aldosterone. Even when this is not the case initially, use of the diuretics, especially on a continuing basis, will usually compel the loss of enough sodium to stimulate the mechanisms for sodium resorption, including aldosterone. So the patient who receives diuretics is likely to have elevated plasma levels of aldosterone.

Thiazide diuretics are believed to act in the distal tubule at a site proximal (upstream) to that for potassium secretion. Thus when sodium resorption is inhibited by these diuretics, additional sodium and tubular fluid are delivered downstream to the potassium-secreting segment of the tubule, which has been primed by aldosterone. Presumably increased resorption of sodium then takes place there (though not enough to nullify the sodium-losing effect of the diuretic). Enhanced sodium resorption at this site increases the negativity of the tubular lumen, promoting the secretion of potassium. The increased flow of tubular fluid carries away secreted potassium, discouraging back-diffusion into the tubular cells. In short, several of the stimuli to potassium secretion listed in Table 8-1 are activated by thiazide diuretics.

Diuretics that act in the loop of Henle will have similar effects on K^+ secretion as well as inhibiting the K^+ resorption that probably takes place in the loop. Otherwise, so far as we know, the mechanisms for potassium resorption in various places along the nephron continue to operate as usual, apparently unconcerned by the influences that have a major impact on the secretion and, ultimately, the excretion of potassium. There are times when different parts of the nephron appear to be working at cross-purposes!

WHO'S IN CHARGE HERE?

In Chapter 4 we discussed the fact that renal excretion of sodium normally responds to, and is in effect controlled by the effective volume of the extracellular fluid or its subdivision, the plasma volume. Though a number of different effector mechanisms in the kidney are involved, the overall effect appears directed toward maintaining the right volume in these fluid compartments.

We might reasonably expect that potassium excretion is similarly controlled by some single important internal factor. If that is the case, we haven't yet learned what it is. It seems more likely that potassium excretion is determined by a number of different influences. If sodium excretion follows the directives of a single boss, potassium excretion appears to be run by a committee.

We know that normal animals and people respond to changes of potassium intake with appropriate adjustments of urinary K^+ excretion. Intracellular potassium concentrations may be the key to this response. Since most of the potassium in the body is sequestered within cells, an increased or decreased potassium intake should have a direct effect on the amount of potassium in the cells, including those in the distal tubule that regulate potassium secretion.

The plasma potassium concentration may also influence K^+ excretion. High levels of circulating potassium stimulate the release of aldosterone from the adrenal glands and thus promote renal excretion of K^+—a seemingly logical homeostatic mechanism. However, aldosterone secretion is also stimulated by way of the renin-angiotensin system in response to depletion of the extracellular fluid volume. In this latter setting it contributes to sodium conservation but may have an adverse effect at times on potassium homeostasis.

As indicated in Table 8-1, a number of factors influence K^+ secretion. We have just discussed how some of these conditions, such as intracellular K^+ concentration and aldosterone secretion, may operate to promote homeostasis for K^+ in the body. It is not so clear how some of other factors mentioned contribute to normal potassium homeostasis. It may be that the renal gain or loss of potassium in response to some of these other influences is not really adaptive from the point of view of potassium homeostasis; rather it may be a necessary trade-off for other adjustments. The urinary losses of potassium that occur in metabolic alkalosis or during an osmotic diuresis may be examples of this. In such cases the urinary loss of K^+, though undesirable, may be less damaging than the possible alternative, such as severe sodium depletion.

SOME UNANSWERED QUESTIONS

Not too many years ago we were far more ignorant about the mechanisms for potassium homeostasis than we are now. It appeared that K^+ balance was an accidental by-product of sodium regulation, though this seemed a strange way to handle such a vital constituent of the body. The direct influence of serum potassium levels on aldosterone secretion is now recognized, as is the relationship between intracellular concentrations of K^+ and its secretion by renal tubules, and the picture is beginning to make more sense. Even so, some pieces are still missing.

For instance, the phenomenon of potassium adaptation is still unexplained. If rats are fed gradually increasing amounts of K^+, they become able to tolerate and excrete enormous quantities that would otherwise be lethal. We still don't know how this adaptation is achieved, though aldosterone appears to be a part of it.

Changes of K^+ excretion in response to alkalosis and acidosis are also very puzzling, since urinary potassium losses may increase in both conditions. It is difficult, to say the least, to explain these observations in terms of the same mechanism.

As more information becomes available about the factors that influence potassium regulation, a more coherent picture of the overall process may emerge.

BIBLIOGRAPHY

G. Malnic, R. M. Klose, and G. Giebisch. Micropuncture study of renal potassium excretion in the rat. *Am. J. Physiol.* 206: 674–686, 1964.

An important and often-quoted laboratory study.

F. S. Wright. Sites and mechanisms of potassium transport along the renal tubule. *Kidney Int.* 11: 415–432, 1977.

A review, with many references. For those really interested in the subject, this entire issue of Kidney International *is devoted to a symposium on potassium homeostasis.*

F. S. Wright and G. Giebisch. Renal potassium transport: Contributions of individual nephron segments and populations. *Am. J. Physiol.* 235: F515–F527, 1978.

Reviews experimental evidence, well-accepted concepts, and unresolved questions.

9
Glomerulopathies

A variety of disease processes may attack the kidneys. Depending on the nature, severity, and duration of the attack, the consequences may range from mild renal dysfunction to marked destruction of renal tissue and loss of renal function. In some situations the causes of disease are recognized, and the mechanisms of damage are understood fairly well. In many cases, however, these remain unknown despite extensive investigation.

Since the causes of renal damage are so often obscure, we are forced to classify renal diseases by their consequences. A renal "disease," therefore, is usually defined by a group of clinical and microscopic findings. Such an approach to classification is not entirely satisfactory. The kidneys can respond to injury only in a limited number of ways, so renal lesions that look alike—and are thus classified as representing the same disease—may actually have been caused by different pathogenic agents or processes. It is also possible that the response of renal tissue to injury is influenced by variables other than the offending agent. In that case, a given insult might product different lesions—that is, different "diseases"—in different kidneys.

Imagine how different our comprehension of lung diseases would be if bacteria and viruses had not been discovered. All pneumonias would then have to be classified not according to their causative agents, but by their clinical and microscopic features. Our understanding of most kidney diseases is at a similar stage today.

Considering our limited knowledge about basic causes, it is not surprising that various investigators have developed differing classifications for renal diseases and coined a host of descriptive terms for them—to the despair of students and the confusion of almost everyone. Yet if renal diseases are to be studied and eventually understood, we must have some system for grouping them on the basis of apparent similarity. The rationale for the classification offered here will be explained shortly. We shall use terminology that is widely accepted, but frequently used alternative names for the same diseases will be mentioned when appropriate.

In this chapter we shall consider renal diseases that are primarily glomerular; that is, they are believed to affect the glomeruli first, even though other renal structures such as tubules and interstitium may also be damaged. As you will see in the next chapter, processes that do not appear to be directed primarily against glomeruli can also result in glomerular damage. It follows that the presence of abnormal glomeruli on microscopic examination does not necessarily indicate a primary glomerular disease.

MECHANISMS OF GLOMERULAR INJURY

Immunologic Injury

Considerable evidence has accumulated over the past two decades to suggest a major role of the immune system in many forms of glomerulonephritis. The most common mechanism thought to be involved in human glomerulonephritis is the deposition of *immune complexes* in glomeruli. These immune complexes, which result from the combination of antigen and antibody molecules, are believed to be formed in the circulation and trapped in glomerular capillary loops in the area of the basement membrane. Evidence to support this theory is derived from both experimental animal studies and observations in man.

Rabbits that have been given a large single injection of a foreign protein will develop *acute serum sickness*—a disorder characterized by inflammatory lesions in their hearts, joints, and kidneys—at a time when complexes of the protein and antibody are detected in the serum. If the rabbits receive smaller but repeated doses of foreign protein, they may develop *chronic serum sickness,* which includes glomerular injury. In both of these models antigen, antibody, and complement components can be demonstrated in glomeruli by immunofluorescence microscopy, a technique for detecting proteins in tissue sections. These proteins are deposited in a granular (resembling small grains) pattern similar to that seen in many human glomerulopathies.

Other animal models also provide strong support for the role of immune-complex deposition in the pathogenesis of glomerular lesions. Animals with chronic viral infections such as lymphocytic choriomeningitis may have circulating complexes of virus and antibody as well as glomerular lesions. New Zealand mice develop a disease resembling systemic lupus erythematosus in which antibodies eluted from the glomeruli react with both nuclear and viral antigens. Thus, it seems that in animals, at least, circulating immune complexes can be trapped in glomeruli and cause glomerulonephritis.

Evidence from the study of humans also suggests that immune-complex deposition is a factor in some glomerular diseases. In many such diseases, circulating immune complexes have been reported. However, detection of these complexes is not an easy or extremely reproducible laboratory procedure. Serum complement levels are depressed in many glomerular diseases (see below), suggesting activation of the complement system by immune complexes and immunoglobulins. Furthermore, components of the complement system are deposited in a granular pattern in the glomeruli of patients with some forms of glomerulonephritis.

Table 9-1. Presumed Antigenic Stimuli in Some Forms of Glomerulonephritis

Antigen	Glomerular Disease
Streptococcal	Acute poststreptococcal glomerulonephritis
Spirochetes	Membranous glomerulonephritis
Malarial organisms	Membranous glomerulonephritis
Hepatitis-B virus	Vasculitis
	Cryoglobulinemic nephritis
	Membranous glomerulonephritis
Gold	Membranous glomerulonephritis
Mercury	Membranous glomerulonephritis
Penicillamine	Membranous glomerulonephritis
Captopril	Membranous glomerulonephritis
Tumor antigens	Membranous glomerulonephritis
Tubular brush border[a]	Membranous glomerulonephritis
Microbes of bacterial endocarditis	Bacterial-endocarditis nephritis
DNA and nuclear proteins	Lupus nephritis

[a]Present in animal models, but not confirmed in human disease.

Systemic lupus erythematosus and bacterial endocarditis are good examples of human diseases in which immune processes result in glomerular injury. Antigenic stimuli are present in the form of nuclear or microbial antigens, and antibodies to these antigens can be demonstrated. In addition, circulating immune complexes and diminished serum complement levels are commonly noted. The glomeruli contain complement as well as complement-fixing immunoglobulins. Nuclear and microbial antigens have also been found in glomeruli on occasion.

In many human glomerular diseases, however, there is no known antigenic stimulus, and the exact pathogenesis remains to be elucidated. Antigens that are related to glomerular diseases, although not always proven to elicit immune-complex-mediated glomerulonephritis, are listed in Table 9-1.

The reasons for localization of immune complexes in glomeruli are not completely understood, but several factors may be important. The generous renal plasma flow as well as the high intracapillary pressure in the glomerulus may predispose it to entrapment of immune complexes. The recent description of complement receptors in human glomerular epithelial cells raises the possibility that these receptors may play a role in immune-complex localization. The size of the circulating immune complex may also determine in part where along the capillary basement membrane it localizes and the type of glomerulonephritis it produces.

But the finding of immunoglobulin deposited in glomeruli needs to be interpreted with caution—it does not prove that immune complexes are responsible for whatever renal disease is present. Immunoglobulins and complement can be detected in the glomeruli of patients with many diseases in which there is little evidence to support an immune-complex pathogenesis. Antigen, specific antibody, and complement must be demonstrable in glomeruli before we can conclude that glomerular deposits are immune complexes and not just incidental deposits of immunoglobulin.

Recent experimental evidence in a model of glomerulonephritis in rats is changing some of our thoughts regarding mechanisms of glomerular injury. Rats injected with renal or tubular tissue or tubular brush-border antigens develop a chronic glomerular disease with electron-dense deposits and immunoglobulins along glomerular basement membranes and also proteinuria. Previously it was felt that the animals made antibody to tubular brush-border antigens and developed circulating immune complexes that then deposited in glomeruli. However, experimental manipulations have demonstrated that antibody to brush-border antigens may react with glomerular sites, forming an in situ immune complex. The antibody to tubular antigens appears to cross-react with glomerular antigens, and the antibody alone can cause the glomerular deposit. The relevance of this to human disease remains uncertain, but it has reawakened our thinking regarding immune mechanisms of injury.

While immune complexes are thought to play a role in up to 70% of human glomerulonephritis, another type of immunological injury may account for less than 5% of human glomerulonephritis. Antibody directed against glomerular basement membrane (GBM) can cause severe renal injury. This has been called *anti-GBM nephritis*. In man, antibody against GBM is associated with a proliferative crescentic glomerulonephritis. If the patient also has intra-alveolar pulmonary hemorrhage, this has been called *Goodpasture's syndrome*. It seems likely that antibody to GBM also has reactivity with alveolar basement membrane in this disease, but there is not a good correlation of antibody levels with pulmonary hemorrhage.

Anti-GBM nephritis can be produced experimentally. First, rat kidney (or GBM) is injected into a rabbit, causing the rabbit to form antibody to rat GBM. When the rabbit serum is injected into rats, the antibodies react with GBM and cause glomerulonephritis. The immunoglobulin can be detected by immunofluorescence techniques, and, in contrast to the granular appearance of immune-complex disease, the fluorescence is located all along the GBM, looks like a ribbon, and is described as *linear*. Linear fluorescence in man is a characteristic finding if anti-GBM antibodies are present, although such fluorescence may be demonstrated occasionally without any identifiable reason.

Immune complexes or specific anti-GBM antibodies probably produce little injury by themselves, requiring mediators to cause damage. The complement system can act as one pathway to glomerular injury. The classical pathway of complement activation is set in motion by complement-fixing immunoglobulins, and the sequential activation of these plasma proteins generates factors that attract polymorphonuclear leukocytes. These leukocytes then release destructive lysosomal enzymes that can damage glomerular structures. While this mechanism seems plausible for such human diseases as acute poststreptococcal glomerulonephritis and lupus nephritis, it may not be the mechanism of injury in all forms of glomerulonephritis, since there are many inflammatory glomerular diseases in which neutrophils are not prominent. In such situations there may be other mediators of inflammation. These may include kinins and cell-mediated immune reactions, though this has not been proved conclusively.

Nonimmune Glomerular Injury

Though immunologic mechanisms of glomerular injury have received major attention in the past two decades, there also appear to be other causes of glomerular damage. These may act alone or in concert with immune processes. Some glomerular problems such as minimal-change disease do not have any proven immunologic basis. Fibrin can be detected in glomeruli in many renal diseases and may play a pathogenetic role. Platelets, which have a shortened life span in some renal diseases, may also initiate glomerular injury through intravascular aggregation. Other factors such as an increased intracapillary pressure within glomeruli, increased or disturbed glomerular blood flow, and malfunction of the phagocytic housekeeping effect of glomerular mesangial cells may eventually prove to be important as well.

APPROACH TO THE DIAGNOSIS OF GLOMERULAR DISEASE

Most textbook discussions of glomerulonephritis begin with specific diseases that cannot be diagnosed accurately without histologic examination of renal tissue. Since this requires renal biopsy, an invasive procedure, it is usually the last part of the evaluation of a patient with possible glomerulonephritis. Thus most descriptions start at the end of the diagnostic road. Therefore, before discussing specific glomerular diseases, we shall try to present an approach to the diagnosis of such problems which begins at the beginning, when the patient first brings his problem to a physician. This approach utilizes available information such as the patient's history, physical findings, urinalysis, total daily protein excretion, and level of renal function as reflected by a measurement of the serum creatinine.

The renal glomerulus may respond to injury in several ways: by decreased filtration, by increased permeability to plasma proteins, by inflammatory changes, or by some combination of these. The characteristics of the glomerular response found in a given patient provide useful information about the type of injury that has occurred.

Decreased glomerular filtration will be apparent if there is a substantial elevation of serum creatinine concentration or if other indicators of renal insufficiency are present. Even in the absence of such evidence, altered glomerular filtration and physical factors within the kidney may lead to sodium and water retention, which in turn can produce edema and hypertension.

Altered glomerular permeability can allow abnormal quantities of plasma protein, mostly albumin, to reach the urine (*proteinuria*). Large amounts of albumin in the urine are often associated with edema, hypoalbuminemia, and sometimes increased blood lipids; this combination of findings is known as the *nephrotic syndrome*. Since the proteinuria appears to be the basic disturbance here and the other abnormalities are not always present, many authors use the term *nephrotic syndrome* to designate any patient whose 24-hour urinary protein excretion exceeds 3.5 g (or correspondingly less in children). Strictly speaking, however, it takes more than one finding to make a syndrome. In this chapter we shall use the term *nephrotic* to refer to a disease (or a person who has the disease) characterized by a urinary protein loss of 3.5 g or more per day, while *nephrotic syndrome* will refer to the combination of findings already described.

Glomerular inflammation is manifested by red blood cells in the urine—*hematuria*—and usually not by white blood cells in the urine—*pyuria*—a finding more often seen with infection of the kidney or bladder. Hematuria is not necessarily indicative of glomerulonephritis, since it may originate anywhere along the urinary tract, including the bladder, and can be caused by infection, tumors, and other inflammation. However, red blood cells entrapped in a protein matrix forming cylindrical *casts* have a more specific meaning. Since casts are formed in renal tubules, red cells within them could not have entered the urine downstream from the kidney. Thus *red-cell casts* in the urine indicate hematuria of renal origin, usually inflammatory glomerulonephritis. Urine that contains many red blood cells is said to have an *active sediment,* especially if casts are also present, because these findings suggest an active inflammatory process in the kidney. The absence of red-cell casts or even hematuria does not rule out glomerulonephritis, however, since proteinuria may be the sole urinary manifestation of the disease. Proteinaceous casts without cells in them, referred to as *hyaline casts,* are often abundant in the urine when large amounts of protein are present.

A glomerular disease can be categorized initially according to whether the patient has a nephrotic pattern, hematuria, or both together. Table 9-2 lists the characteristics of various glomerulopathies at the time of initial presentation. For purposes of simplicity, diseases are listed under the heading usually associated with them, but it is possible that occasionally they may appear under another heading. For example, membranous glomerulonephritis usually produces a nephrotic picture, and less than 10 red blood cells per high-power field (RBC/hpf) are seen on urinalysis (pure nephrotic disease). However, occasionally hematuria and red blood cell casts, an active sediment, may be noted. Diseases that are often variable in their presentation are listed under two headings.

This classification enables us to narrow the spectrum of possible diagnoses to a particular group of conditions. Other information such as serum complement levels, the presence or absence of renal insufficiency, physical findings, and the patient's history may then help us to focus on a specific

Table 9-2. Characteristics of Glomerular Diseases at Presentation

Pure Nephrotic Pattern	Mixed Nephrotic and Hematuria	Hematuria Non-nephrotic
Minimal change[a]	Systemic lupus (diffuse	Acute poststreptococcal[a,b]
Focal sclerosing[a]	proliferative, mem-	Recurrent hematuria[a]
Membranous[a]	branous)[b]	Crescentic (including
Diabetes mellitus	Membranoproliferative[b]	Goodpasture's syn-
Amyloidosis	Endocarditis[b]	drome)
	Cryoglobulinemia[b]	Vasculitis
	Anaphylactoid purpura[a]	Hemolytic uremic syn-
		drome
		Thrombotic throm-
		bocytopenic purpura
		Hereditary nephritis
		Systemic lupus (focal, mes-
		angial)[b]
		Anaphylactoid purpura[a]

[a]Not usually associated with renal insufficiency at presentation.

[b]Depressed serum complement levels.

Hematuria = > 10 red blood cells/hpf on urinalysis

Nephrotic pattern = > 3.5 g/day protein in urine

disease within the group. For example, if an elderly person appears with pure nephrotic disease (less than 10 RBCs/hpf on urinalysis), cardiomegaly, orthostatic hypotension, and an elevated serum creatinine level—reflecting a decreased glomerular filtration rate—we can be suspicious of amyloidosis. Of the diseases listed in Table 9-2 that have a pure nephrotic pattern, the two commonly associated with renal insufficiency at presentation are amyloidosis and diabetes mellitus. Since for practical purposes diabetic nephropathy doesn't exist without clinical diabetes, we can exclude this diagnosis. Minimal-change disease and focal sclerosis (see below) are more common in children, but can be found in adults. The enlarged heart and orthostatic changes may be related to infiltration of the heart and blood vessels by amyloid. The actual diagnosis in our theoretical patient may not be amyloidosis, but at least the schema has made us think of this possibility. The reader should be aware that Table 9-2 does not include interstitial diseases that may be associated with hematuria.

Individual glomerulopathies are listed in Tables 9-3, 9-4, and 9-5 and will be discussed briefly. Before we describe the clinicopathologic characteristics of separate glomerulopathies, a brief introduction to histologic terminology is in order.

Proliferation refers to an increase in cells in the glomerulus regardless of origin.

Sclerosis refers to eosinophilic material in the glomerulus. It is used loosely to describe an increase in mesangial matrix, collagen, or even large insudative lesions underneath the capillary basement membrane. (The *mesangium* is the supporting structure of the glomerulus that holds the capillaries together. An *insudative lesion* is a seepage of protein-rich material into a tissue.)

Focal means that some glomeruli, but not all, are involved with a process. *Generalized* means that all glomeruli are involved. *Segmental* means that part of a glomerulus is involved and *diffuse* refers to the entire glomerulus. On electron microscopic examination, deposits are described by their location. *Subendothelial deposits* are between the endothelial cell and the capillary basement membrane, *intramembranous* are within the basement membrane, and *subepithelial deposits* are outside the basement membrane underneath the visceral epithelial cell. A *crescent* is a sickle-shaped collection of epithelial cells along the inside wall of Bowman's capsule. It is external to glomerular capillaries and may compress them.

SPECIFIC TYPES OF GLOMERULONEPHRITIS

PURE NEPHROTIC DISEASE (See Table 9-3)

Minimal-Change Disease

(Synonyms: idiopathic nephrotic syndrome, lipoid nephrosis, "nil" disease, foot-process disease.)

Minimal-change disease is a disorder, more common in young children, that produces the nephrotic syndrome, usually without hematuria, hypertension, or renal functional impairment. It accounts for over 80% of cases of nephrotic syndrome of children, but it also occurs in adults of any age. Most cases occur between the ages of one and five years. It may follow upper respiratory tract infections or prophylactic immunizations and has been associated with Hodgkin's disease. Striking edema or even anasarca (massive generalized fluid accumulation) may be present. The urine contains a large amount of albumin, and blood lipids are usually elevated.

Treatment with corticosteroids leads to cessation of proteinuria in 60 to 90% of patients, though relapses may occur. Cyclophosphamide decreases the relapse rate and can prolong remission, but toxicity precludes initial or prolonged use. The prognosis is good because renal failure rarely if ever develops.

Pathogenesis and Histology

The pathogenesis remains unknown, although unproven theories have been proposed. It does not appear to be mediated by known immunologic mechanisms. By light microscopic examination, glomeruli appear normal (Fig. 9-1)

Table 9-3. Outline of Glomerular Diseases Characterized by a Pure Nephrotic Pattern

Disease	Age	Urine Sediment	Proteinuria	Renal Function at Presentation[a]	Serum C3[a]	Serum C4[a]	Comment	Therapy	Prognosis
Minimal-change disease	Children more common, but any age	Inactive	++++	Nl	Nl	Nl	Can be associated with Hodgkin's disease	Prednisone; cyclophosphamide for nonresponders	Good
Focal sclerosing glomerulonephritis	Children more common, but any age	Inactive	++++	Usually Nl	Nl	Nl		None	Renal failure in 70–80%
Membranous glomerulonephritis	Adults usually	Inactive	+++	Usually Nl	Nl	Nl	Associated with drugs, mercury, gold, hepatitis-B, carcinoma	Prednisone	20% remission; renal failure in 80%; slowly progressive
Diabetic glomerulopathy	Adults	Inactive	+++	→	Nl	Nl	Multisystem disease	None	Very poor
Amyloidosis	Adults usually	Inactive	+++	→	Nl	Nl	Multisystem disease	None	Very poor

[a]Nl = normal.

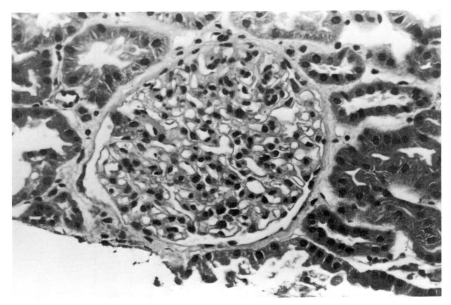

Figure 9-1. A glomerulus from a patient with minimal-change disease. No abnormalities are noted. (Hematoxylin and eosin stain ×320)

except for minimal swelling of glomerular epithelial cells and occasionally slight prominence of mesangial cells and matrix. By immunofluorescence microscopy, only minimal glomerular deposition of immunoglobulins and complement components is seen in some cases. By electron microscopy, foot processes are lost, and the visceral epithelial cells appear swollen. No electron-dense deposits are present.

Focal Sclerosing Glomerulonephritis

This diagnosis is based on the histologic demonstration of segmental sclerosis of glomeruli. Unfortunately, it probably does not represent a single disease entity, but rather a renal response to various injuries. The histologic finding of focal glomerulosclerosis in a young patient with nephrotic syndrome portends a poor prognosis and therefore is helpful in planning therapy and prognostication. The vast majority of young nephrotic patients with focal glomerular sclerosis will advance to renal failure, unresponsive to corticosteroid or other immunosuppressive forms of therapy. Patients present in a manner similar to patients with minimal-change disease, but the relationship between these two conditions remains controversial. It is unknown whether nonresponsive minimal-change disease can evolve into renal failure with glomerular sclerosis, or whether renal failure occurs only in those who have had undetected glomerular sclerosis from the beginning.

Pathogenesis and Histology

The pathogenesis is unknown but is not felt to be mediated by known immunologic mechanisms. Focal glomerular sclerosis with typical histologic lesions has a high rate of recurrence in renal transplants, suggesting a host pathogenetic factor. By light microscopy, segmental hyaline sclerosis is noted with large insudative hyaline deposits in a subendothelial location. These lesions have a predilection for glomeruli located near the medulla of the kidney. Immunofluorescence studies reveal glomerular IgM and complement components in a focal segmental pattern. Electron microscopic examination will reveal large electron-dense deposits, occasionally with vacuoles, which correspond to the insudative lesions seen on light microscopy. The basement membrane is wrinkled in sclerotic areas.

Membranous Glomerulonephritis

(Synonym: membranous nephropathy)

Membranous glomerulonephritis is characterized by subepithelial deposits on the basement membrane of glomerular capillaries without an increase in cellularity. Most patients have moderate to heavy proteinuria and the nephrotic syndrome. Hematuria can occur, especially in males, but is not a prominent feature. Membranous nephropathy may appear at any age but is more common after childhood, being the most common cause of nephrotic syndrome in adults. It has occurred in patients being treated with penicillamine, gold, trimethadone, and mercury. It has also been associated with hepatitis-B virus infections, quartan malaria, syphilis, sarcoidosis, and schistosomiasis, as well as various carcinomata. The vast majority of patients with membranous glomerulonephritis will progress slowly to renal failure, although up to 20% may experience spontaneous remissions. Treatment is controversial, but recent controlled studies suggest that corticosteroids retard progressive renal failure.

Pathogenesis and Histology

The pathogenesis is unknown, but the association with antigenic agents and similar histologic alterations in animal models suggest a process involving immune complexes. While there is much to be said for this view, normal serum complement levels do not support it, and the evidence for circulating immune complexes has been conflicting. The glomeruli are normocellular by light microscopy with normal to very thickened capillary basement membranes. On silver-stained sections "spikes" can be seen protruding out from capillary walls (Fig. 9-2). These spikes represent basement membrane protruding between subepithelial deposits. In late stages of the disease there is significant glomerular sclerosis. By immunofluorescence microscopy fine granular deposits of immunoglobulins and complement are seen along glomerular capillary walls (Fig. 9-3).

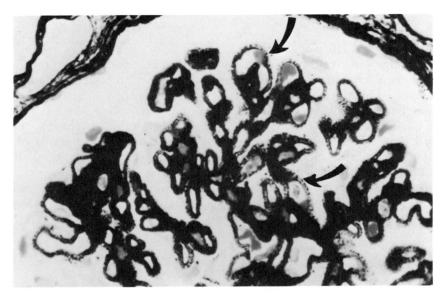

Figure 9-2. Glomerulus processed with a silver stain demonstrating "spikes" (arrows) of basement membrane protruding around subepithelial deposits. These capillary spikes are seen typically in membranous nephropathy. (×400)

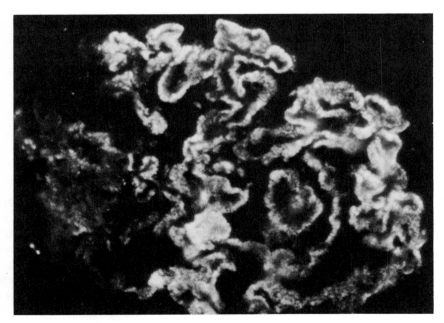

Figure 9-3. Immunofluorescence microscopy demonstrating granular deposits of IgG along glomerular capillaries in a patient with membranous nephropathy. "Granules" correspond to subepithelial deposits noted on electron microscopic examination. (×400)

134

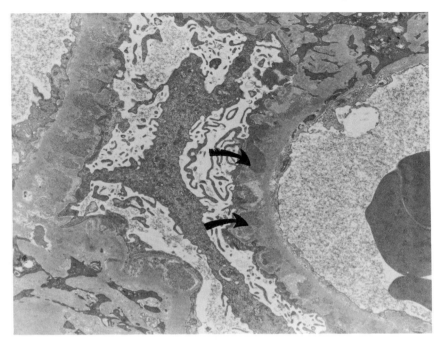

Figure 9-4. Electron-dense deposits (arrows) along the outside of a glomerular capillary typical of advanced membranous nephropathy.

Electron microscopic examination reveals the subepithelial electron-dense deposits that are characteristic of the disease (Fig. 9-4).

Diabetic Nephropathy

The kidney is involved in the vascular disease associated with long-standing carbohydrate intolerance. Renal involvement in patients with juvenile-onset, insulin-dependent diabetes mellitus is more common than in those with the adult-onset form of the disease, although it may occur in both types. Patients with diabetic renal disease make up a growing proportion of those with end-stage renal failure receiving dialysis, and they account for up to 15% of renal transplants done in some centers.

The renal lesion usually occurs after 15 to 20 years of insulin dependence and is almost always associated with vascular involvement of the eye (retinopathy). Other blood vessels and the nervous system are also frequently involved. The most common presentation is proteinuria with the nephrotic syndrome and hypertension. Hematuria can occur but is not a prominent feature. Once proteinuria and hypertension are present, the prognosis is very poor, with progression to death or renal failure in three years the rule.

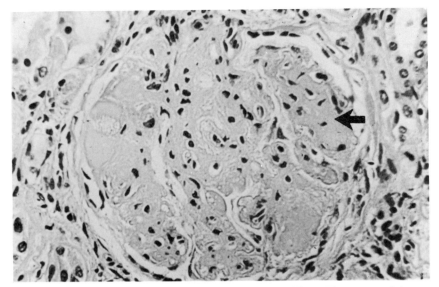

Figure 9-5. Glomerulus from a patient with diabetes mellitus. The mesangial areas are thickened by "sclerotic" material (arrow). (Hematoxylin and eosin stain ×320)

Pathogenesis and Histology

The renal lesion in all probability is related to the widespread microvascular disease. The exact pathogenesis of these vascular lesions is not known, but hyperglycemia seemingly plays a role. Light microscopic examination will reveal diffuse and nodular glomerular sclerosis and hyaline sclerosis of arterioles (Fig. 9-5). Hyaline lesions in the afferent and efferent arterioles of the same glomerulus are typical of diabetes mellitus. Insudative PAS-positive lesions can be seen in glomerular capillary loops (fibrin cap) or Bowman's capsule (capsular drop). These lesions are characteristic but not necessarily diagnostic of diabetes mellitus.

Immunofluorescence studies will occasionally demonstrate immunoglobulins, complement, and fibrinogen in vascular and glomerular insudative lesions, but widespread granular deposits are not seen. Frequently IgG will be present in a linear pattern along glomerular and tubular basement membranes. This is thought to reflect a nonimmunologic accumulation of IgG and does not represent anti-GBM antibodies. Electron microscopy will demonstrate glomerular capillary thickening, sclerosis, and large subendothelial insudative lesions.

Amyloidosis

Amyloidosis accounts for up to 12% of cases of nephrotic syndrome in adulthood. Primary amyloidosis or secondary amyloidosis both can involve the kidney. The amyloid protein from patients with primary or myeloma-

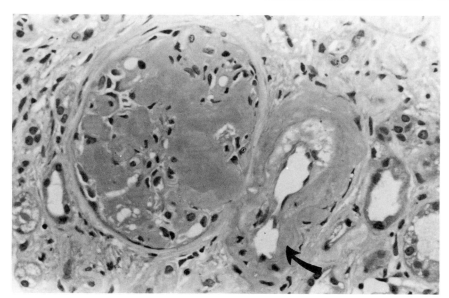

Figure 9-6. Glomerulus and renal artery from a patient with amyloidosis. Amyloid appears eosinophilic on light microscopic examination and can occasionally resemble diabetic nephropathy. Note material present in vessel wall (arrow). (Hematoxylin and eosin stain ×250)

related amyloidosis consists mainly of fragments of immunoglobulin light chains. In secondary amyloidosis a nonimmunoglobulin protein called AA protein constitutes the major component of amyloid fibrils. Patients with amyloidosis usually have proteinuria and only minimal hematuria. Renal failure may be present initially or may subsequently develop, but the prognosis is very poor. There is no successful treatment other than treatment of the primary disease in the case of secondary amyloidosis.

Pathogenesis and Histology
The renal disease appears to be secondary to deposition of amyloid protein within the kidney. By light microscopy, amyloid is seen in glomeruli as an acellular eosinophilic substance in mesangial areas and along capillary loops (Fig. 9-6). It may also be noted in vessel walls and interstitium. Special stains such as Congo red, sirius red, crystal violet or thioflavin-T will aid in the diagnosis. Electron microscopy shows that the deposits contain fibrils with characteristics specific for amyloid (Fig. 9-7).

NEPHROTIC PATTERN WITH HEMATURIA (See Table 9-4)

Patients with diseases discussed below commonly have both significant proteinuria and hematuria when they first present themselves to a physician.

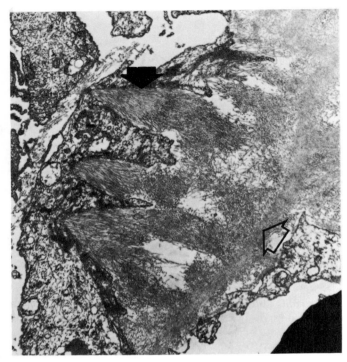

Figure 9-7. Amyloid fibrils (dark arrow) in a glomerulus examined with an electron microscope. Capillary basement membrane is noted by open arrow.

Hematuria may be obvious upon looking at the urine (gross hematuria) or detectable only upon microscopic examination. It is also possible, but less likely, that a patient with one of these diseases may have either pure nephrotic syndrome or hematuria with only minimal proteinuria.

Systemic Lupus Erythematosus (SLE)

SLE is a multisystem disease. Joints, skin, hematologic, cardiovascular, pulmonary, and central nervous systems may be involved in addition to the kidney. Young adult women are most susceptible to SLE, with females being affected seven times as frequently as males. Renal involvement in these patients may vary from only minimal hematuria to nephrotic syndrome or renal failure. Physical examination may be helpful in making the diagnosis, since a typical rash over the cheeks may be seen as well as other skin or joint manifestations. Laboratory studies are very useful in establishing the diagnosis. LE cells may be found, and antinuclear antibodies are almost always present in the serum. Leukopenia or thrombocytopenia may be detected, and a hemolytic anemia mediated by antibodies to red blood cells may also be

Table 9-4. Outline of Glomerular Diseases Characterized by a Nephrotic Pattern with Hematuria

Disease	Age	Urine Sediment	Proteinuria	Renal Function at Presentation[a]	Serum C3[a]	Serum C4[a]	Comment	Therapy	Prognosis
Systemic lupus erythematosus	Young adult, usually female	Active	+++	Nl usually	↓	↓	Multisystem disease	Prednisone ± immunosuppressives	Often responds to therapy
Membranoproliferative glomerulonephritis	Young usually	Active	+++	Nl or ↓	often ↓	often ↓	C3 nephritic factor in serum of some Can recur in allografts	Dipyridamole, warfarin (?) Long-term prednisone (?)	Renal failure in 70–90%
Glomerulonephritis with bacterial endocarditis	Any age	Active	++	↓	↓	↓	Valvular heart disease	Antibiotics; surgery	Good if treated early
Mixed cryoglobulinemia	Elderly	Active	+++	Variable	↓	↓	Liver disease common; related to hepatitis-B(?)	Immunosuppressive therapy	Poor, though improvement may occur
Anaphylactoid purpura	Children usually	Active	++	Nl usually	Nl	Nl	GI tract, skin, joints involved	None	10% progress to renal failure

[a]Nl = normal.

present. Serum complement levels of both C3 and C4 components are usually decreased when the kidney is involved.

Treatment with corticosteroids is beneficial in SLE with renal involvement. Whether immunosuppressive agents such as azathioprine or cyclophosphamide add any benefit to corticosteroid therapy is not definitely known at this time, but added improvement, if present, is not striking. The prognosis of patients with SLE depends on the organ systems affected, with involvement of the kidneys or central nervous system having a worse prognosis. The type of renal involvement (see below) also can affect the outcome. In general, the more proliferative the glomerular lesion, the worse the prognosis. Ten-year survival figures may range from 50 to 90% in treated patients.

Pathogenesis and Histology

SLE is considered a prototype of human immune-complex disease. Immune complexes can be detected in serum and glomeruli. Native DNA and antibodies against it appear to be of major importance. Serum complement levels are depressed, reflecting activation of the classical complement pathway, and mediators of glomerular injury such as polymorphonuclear leukocytes are commonly seen in damaged glomeruli.

By light microscopy there are several different histologic patterns. In the past it was believed that the histologic pattern shown by a patient would almost always remain the same, but recent studies suggest that there may be a change of histologic pattern in up to 30% of patients. The least severe pattern is *mesangial proliferative* with only a minimal generalized increase in mesangial cells. *Focal proliferative lupus nephritis* has a focal and segmental increase in glomerular cellularity. Basement membranes are generally normal in nonproliferative areas of glomeruli. *Diffuse proliferative lupus nephritis* (Fig. 9-8) refers to more generalized proliferation with basement membrane thickening to form so-called wire loops. There may be nuclear disruption in glomerular cells with necrosis and sclerosis. The interstitium may be fibrotic and infiltrated with mononuclear cells. Hematoxylin bodies are lilac-colored areas in the cytoplasm of glomerular cells, but despite textbook descriptions to the contrary, they are not specific and too difficult to find to be helpful in the diagnosis of SLE. *Membranous lupus nephritis* is histologically very similar to idiopathic membranous glomerulonephritis.

By immunofluorescence microscopy, lupus nephritis is distinguished by the number of different immunoglobulins and complement components seen in glomeruli. In addition to IgG (Fig. 9-9), C3 and C4, IgA, IgM, IgE, fibrin, and properdin may be deposited in a granular fashion in glomeruli. Extraglomerular immunoglobulin and complement may also be noted along Bowman's capsule and tubular basement membrane in a granular distribution.

Electron-dense deposits may be seen in a subepithelial location or may also be located within basement membranes or in mesangial areas. The "wire loops" are composed of large subendothelial deposits (Fig. 9-10). Deposits occasionally have a "finger print" crystalline nature. Typical, but not confined

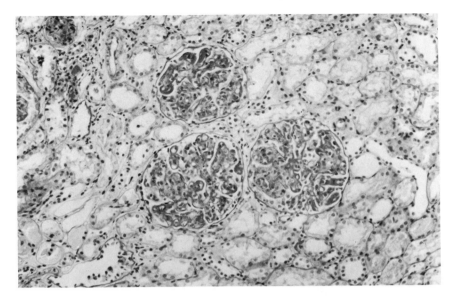

Figure 9-8. Three glomeruli from a patient with diffuse proliferative lupus nephritis. Glomerular cellularity is increased and capillary walls are thickened. (Hematoxylin and eosin ×125)

to SLE, is the finding of microtubular structures within glomerular endothelial cytoplasm (Fig. 9-11).

Membranoproliferative Glomerulonephritis

(Synonyms: mesangiocapillary glomerulonephritis, hypocomplementemic glomerulonephritis)

Membranoproliferative glomerulonephritis has been categorized only in the past two decades. Affected patients are usually young, have proteinuria and hematuria, and commonly are hypertensive. Although two histologic types are described, they are associated with similar clinical characteristics. Serum complement levels are depressed in 80% of patients, although values can fluctuate. Both C3 and C4 levels are low in type I, while C4 levels may be normal in type II. Renal failure will almost always progress to end-stage renal disease over a period of years. Fifty percent of patients will die or require dialysis after 10 to 12 years. No specific treatment is available; however, anticoagulants and antiplatelet agents may slow progression of the disease.

Pathogenesis and Histology

Research into the pathogenesis of membranoproliferative glomerulonephritis was active in the past decade. Unfortunately, as is commonly the case, many questions remain unanswered, and new questions have arisen. Briefly, our

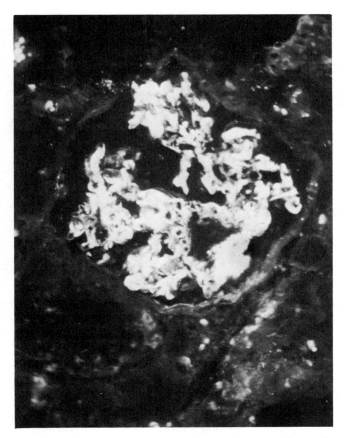

Figure 9-9. Immunofluorescent pattern of IgG deposition in a glomerulus of a patient with systemic lupus erythematosus. (×400)

Figure 9-10. Capillary loop of a glomerulus in lupus nephritis. Large electron-dense deposits are seen on the inside of the basement membrane (U-shaped arrow); these give the capillary a wire-loop appearance on light microscopy. There is also a single subepithelial deposit (slightly curved arrow).

Figure 9-11. Electron micrograph demonstrating microtubular particles in glomerular endothelial cell cytoplasm (arrows). These particles are commonly noted in lupus nephritis.

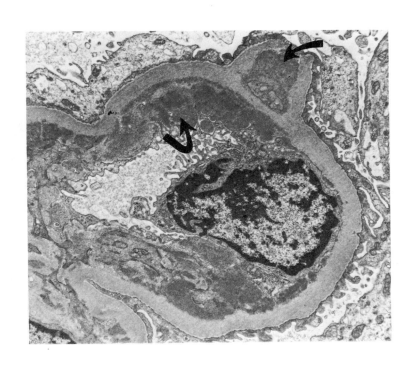

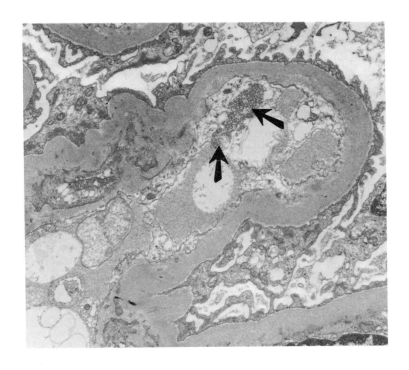

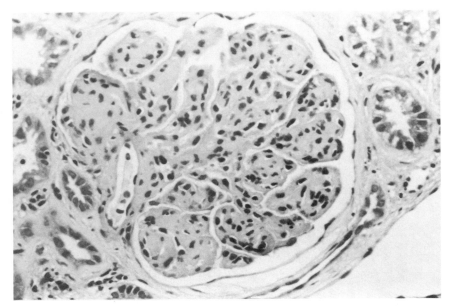

Figure 9-12. Membranoproliferative glomerulonephritis. Note increase in cellularity, lobular appearance and increase in mesangial matrix. (Hematoxylin and eosin ×400)

current understanding suggests that type I may be mediated by immune complexes, although no antigenic stimulus has been identified. Type II is often associated with the presence in the serum of a 7S gamma globulin which protects a stimulator of the alternative complement pathway; this leads to alternate-pathway activation. This protein was initially called C3 nephritic factor. No actual "nephritic role" has yet been described, however, since activation of the alternate pathway doesn't produce renal disease in animal models. It is possible that defects in complement function lead to abnormal handling of immune complexes and resultant renal disease. By light microscopy the glomeruli are enlarged with both cellular proliferation and basement membrane thickening (Fig. 9-12). Polymorphonuclear leukocytes may be noted in glomeruli. Basement membranes may also be split. Mesangial areas may be thickened, giving the glomeruli a lobular appearance.

The glomeruli will contain granular deposits of immunoglobulins, complement, and properdin demonstrated by immunofluorescence microscopy (Fig. 9-13). Electron microscopic examination will delineate the two types. *Type I* has subendothelial and mesangial deposits with thickened and split or reduplicated glomerular capillary basement membranes (Fig. 9-14). Mesangial-cell cytoplasm will extend out along capillary loops between the split basement membrane. *Type II* has electron-dense deposits *within* the basement membrane (Fig. 9-15). These deposits may also be detected in

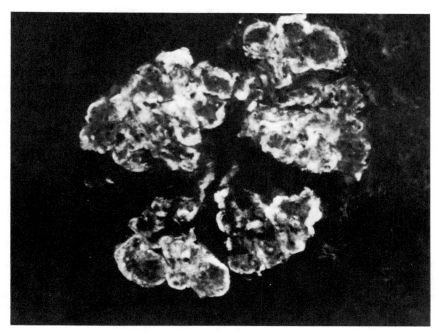

Figure 9-13. Immunofluorescence microscopy of IgM in a glomerulus of a patient with membranoproliferative glomerulonephritis. Note large peripheral immunoglobulin deposits. (×400)

tubular basement membranes. This type has also been called *electron-dense-deposit disease.*

Glomerulonephritis Associated with Endocarditis

The major damage to the kidney in bacterial endocarditis is caused by immunologic mechanisms, not by septic microemboli. The characteristic setting is in a patient with proven or suspected endocarditis. Hematuria and proteinuria are usually both present. Serum complement levels of C3 and C4 are depressed, and rheumatoid factor is commonly present. The renal disease will usually improve with treatment of the underlying infective process.

Pathogenesis and Histology

Glomerular disease is related to the deposition of immune complexes. There is no characteristic histologic lesion; focal and diffuse glomerular proliferation may both be present as well as proliferative crescents on occasion. Immunoglobulins and complement are seen in a granular pattern in glomeruli by immunofluorescence microscopy, and subendothelial, subepithelial, and mesangial deposits may be noted by electron microscopy.

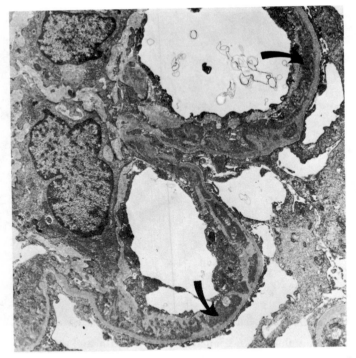

Figure 9-14. Electron micrograph of type I membranoproliferative glomerulonephritis. Subendothelial electron-dense deposits (arrows) are present with basement membrane on both sides of them. This causes the appearance of a "tram-track" on light microscopic examination.

Cryoglobulinemia

Cryoglobulins are serum proteins that precipitate at 4°C. Small amounts may be associated with circulating immune complexes. Larger amounts of cryoglobulins are found in a rare syndrome called *essential cryoglobulinemia* that is usually accompanied by renal disease. The cryoproteins are usually immunoglobulins. Many of these patients have antibodies against the hepatitis-B virus, which may play a role in the pathogenesis. A vasculitis is present in skin, kidney, and occasionally bowel. C3 and C4 complement levels are depressed, and rheumatoid factor is present in the serum. There is no typical histologic pattern of renal involvement, with focal proliferation and a membranoproliferative glomerulonephritis seen in addition to patchy vasculitis. Treatment with immunosuppressive agents may help, but the prognosis is very poor.

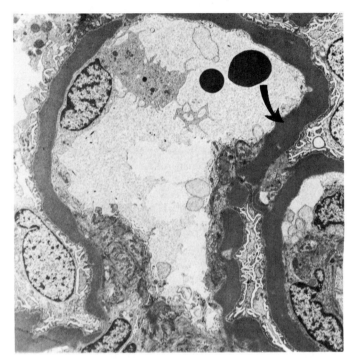

Figure 9-15. Electron micrograph of type II membranoproliferative glomerulone-phritis. Very dense deposits (arrow) are noted within glomerular capillary basement membranes. Some of these are sausage-shaped.

Anaphylactoid Purpura

(Synonym: Henoch-Schönlein purpura)

Anaphylactoid purpura is a syndrome characterized by skin rash, gastrointestinal, musculoskeletal, and renal involvement. Children and young adults are most commonly affected, but it can be present at any age. Skin lesions are urticarial followed by purpuric lesions, usually located below the waist. The renal disease is manifest by hematuria with or without significant proteinuria. Prolonged nephrotic syndrome is unusual. The renal disease is usually self-limited, but progression to end-stage renal disease may occur in about 10% of patients. Recurrent hematuria may continue for years. Serum complement levels are normal.

Pathogenesis and Histology

It is currently believed that anaphylactoid purpura is mediated by circulating immune complexes, but not all features of the disease fit this hypothesis. By light microscopy there is no specific alteration of glomeruli. Diffuse mesangial proliferation, focal proliferation, and crescentic nephritis may be present. Immunofluorescence microscopy reveals most of the immunoglobulins, including IgA and C3 complement. Electron-dense deposits are seen in subendothelial and mesangial areas.

HEMATURIA WITHOUT NEPHROTIC PATTERN (See Table 9-5)

Heavy proteinuria or nephrotic syndrome are usually not associated with these conditions but may occur occasionally.

Acute Poststreptococcal Glomerulonephritis (APSGN)

APSGN follows infection with one of several strains of *nephritogenic* group A streptococci. The initial infection may involve the skin or pharynx. One or two weeks following infection the urine will appear red or brown, and edema and hypertension are commonly present. Children are most commonly affected, but APSGN may occur at any age. Throat cultures will be positive for streptococci in less than 50% of those appearing with nephritis, but many will have elevated antistreptolysin-O (ASO) titers. Serum C3 levels are depressed from 2 to 12 weeks but usually return to normal levels. Most patients with APSGN have only a mild degree of renal impairment from which early and complete recovery is the rule. On rare occasions, however, there is a severe degree of acute renal insufficiency that may evolve into end-stage renal disease. It has been stated that there may also be slow progression to chronic renal failure in some patients, but this appears to be uncommon. Treatment should be directed at the infection, edema, and hypertension.

Pathogenesis and Histology

APSGN represents an immune-complex disease similar in some respects to acute serum sickness, described earlier in the section on mechanisms of glomerular injury. Immune complexes consisting of streptococcal antigens and antibodies against them are deposited in the kidney with ensuing glomerulonephritis. The transient hypocomplementemia supports this concept.

Glomerular lesions by light microscopy are generalized and diffuse. The glomeruli are enlarged with variable amounts of proliferation of intrinsic glomerular cells. Polymorphonuclear leukocytes are frequently present in glomeruli as well. Basement membranes are only minimally thickened, but subepithelial deposits may be noted. In rapidly progressive disease proliferative crescents are common.

By immunofluorescence microscopy, IgG, C3, and occasionally properdin are seen in a granular fashion along peripheral capillary loops. Subepithelial electron-dense humps or deposits with a haystacklike appearance are seen on

Table 9-5. Outline of Glomerular Diseases Characterized by Hematuria without a Nephrotic Pattern

Disease	Age	Urine Sediment	Proteinuria	Renal Function at Presentation[a]	Serum C3[a]	Serum C4[a]	Comment	Therapy	Prognosis
Acute poststreptococcal	Childhood	Active	+ / ++	Slight ↓	↓ for 2–12 weeks	↓ to Nl	Sodium retention and hypertension	Penicillin, diuretics, antihypertensives	Good; progression to chronic renal disease in a few
Recurrent hematuria	Young adults, male > female	Active	±	Nl	Nl	Nl	↑IgA in 50%	Observe	15% progress to renal failure
Crescentic glomerulonephritis (including Goodpasture's)	Young males > females	Active	+ / ++	→	Nl	Nl	Pulmonary hemorrhage in some; Can recur in allografts	Plasmapheresis and immunosuppressive?	Poor; 80% renal failure
Vasculitis	Any age	Active	+	→	Nl	Nl	Multisystem disease	Prednisone	Fair; renal disease may respond to prednisone
Hemolytic uremic syndrome and thrombotic thrombocytopenic purpura	Children, adults	Active	±	→	Nl	Nl	Microangiopathy, hypertension	Antiplatelet drugs, plasmapheresis	Poor for TTP Better for HUS
Hereditary nephritis	Young adults	Active	+ / ++	Variable	Nl	Nl	Autosomal dominant ↓ hearing	None	Renal failure in males

[a]Nl = normal

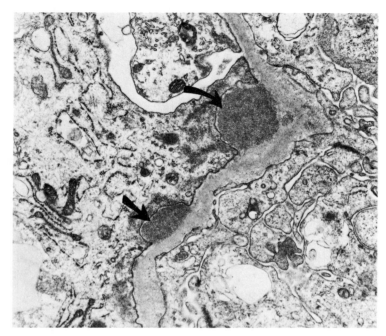

Figure 9-16. Electron micrograph demonstrating subepithelial "humps" or electron-dense deposits (arrows) in acute poststreptococcal glomerulonephritis. An epithelial cell is to the left of the basement membrane, and a swollen endothelial cell is to the right.

electron microscopy (Fig. 9-16). Polymorphonuclear leukocytes may be seen located near the deposits, and breaks in the basement membrane may occur.

Recurrent Hematuria Syndromes

(Synonyms: benign recurrent hematuria, IgA nephropathy, Berger's disease)

Benign recurrent hematuria and IgA nephropathy have very similar clinical pictures. Young patients are most commonly affected, with a strong male predominance. Hematuria may be either gross or microscopic. It commonly occurs with an upper respiratory infection or gastrointestinal illness. Unlike poststreptococcal glomerulonephritis, however, the hematuria is coincident with the illness rather than following it. Proteinuria and nephrotic syndrome are uncommon. Serum complement levels are normal, but IgA levels may be increased. As the name implies, however, frequent repeated episodes of hematuria may occur over many years. Renal failure may occur eventually in up to 15% of patients with IgA nephropathy, but less frequently in patients with benign recurrent hematuria. There is no specific treatment.

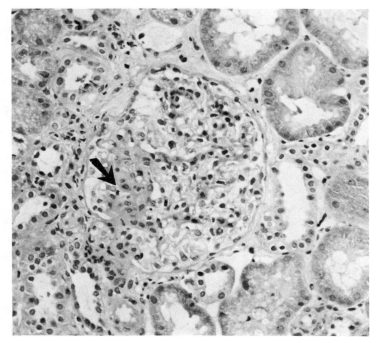

Figure 9-17. Segmental proliferative glomerular lesion in a patient with IgA nephropathy. Arrow denotes proliferative segment. (Hematoxylin and eosin ×250)

Pathogenesis and Histology

The pathogenesis is unknown. Theories that these are immune-complex disorders are as yet unproven. The glomerular lesions are variable. Glomeruli may be normal or demonstrate a diffuse or focal segmental mesangial proliferation (Fig. 9-17). The mesangial areas may also be widened. Glomeruli in benign recurrent hematuria will have no immunoglobulin deposition by immunofluorescent studies. IgA nephropathy, by contrast, will have IgA (Fig. 9-18), IgG, IgM, C3, properdin, and fibrin deposition in mesangial areas. Electron microscopy will reveal only minimal mesangial widening in benign recurrent hematuria, while electron-dense deposits will be noted in mesangial areas with IgA nephropathy (Fig. 9-19).

Crescentic Glomerulonephritis

(Synonyms: Goodpasture's syndrome, rapidly progressive glomerulonephritis)

Proliferative glomerular crescents may be present in association with many glomerular diseases such as lupus nephritis, APSGN, membranoproliferative glomerulonephritis, and others. When glomerular crescents are present, the

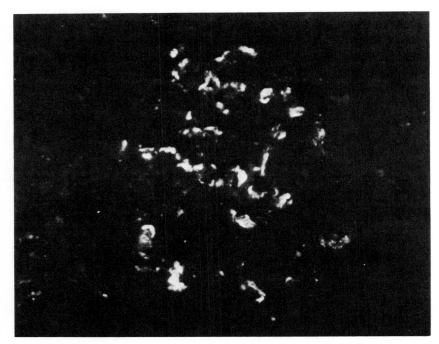

Figure 9-18. Immunofluorescence microscopy of a glomerulus with mesangial deposits of IgA from a patient with IgA nephropathy. (×400)

prognosis is worse. Proliferative crescents are the most striking abnormality in an entity called *crescentic glomerulonephritis.* Some but not all of these patients will have evidence of antibodies against glomerular basement membrane. Goodpasture described a patient with pulmonary hemorrhage and crescentic nephritis, and this association now bears his name. Crescentic nephritis is commonly rapidly progressive, with renal failure occurring in a matter of weeks or months. Pulmonary hemorrhage, which can be severe and life-threatening, will be present in a minority of patients with crescentic nephritis. There is no other evidence of systemic involvement. Males are affected seven times as frequently as females.

Serum complement levels are normal. Antibodies against glomerular basement membrane may be detected in the serum. There is no specific therapy. Prednisone may decrease the pulmonary hemorrhage but has little apparent effect on the renal disease. Plasmapheresis is currently in vogue but has not stood the test of time or controlled prospective studies.

Pathogenesis and Histology
In those cases where fluorescent-antibody techniques show a *linear* deposition of IgG along glomerular capillaries, there is reason to believe that antibodies directed against glomerular basement membrane are responsible for the

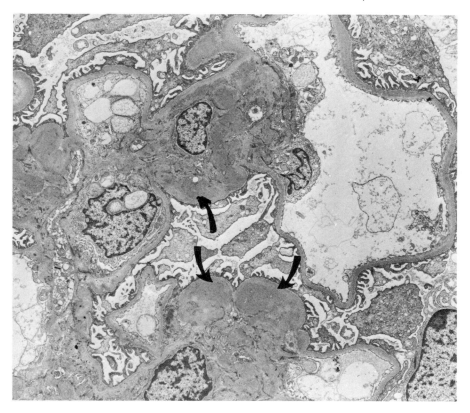

Figure 9-19. Electron micrograph of a glomerulus from a patient with IgA nephropathy. Electron-dense deposits (arrows) are noted in mesangial areas.

disease. These antibodies may cross-react with alveolar basement membrane to cause pulmonary hemorrhage. In cases where the IgG deposits in glomeruli have a granular pattern, or where there are no demonstrable IgG deposits, the pathogenesis is unknown.

Proliferative crescents are seen by light microscopy (Fig. 9-20). Segmental glomerular necrosis and hemorrhage into Bowman's space may also be present. There is usually extensive interstitial disease. Linear deposition of IgG in glomeruli is noted by immunofluorescence microscopy in most cases (Fig. 9-21). Fibrin is commonly seen in areas of crescent formation. Perforations of glomerular basement membranes may be demonstrated, but electron-dense deposits are usually not seen by electron microscopy.

Vasculitis

The term *vasculitis* includes a variety of vascular diseases with systemic effects. *Polyarteritis nodosa* involves larger vessels causing aneurysmal dilatation,

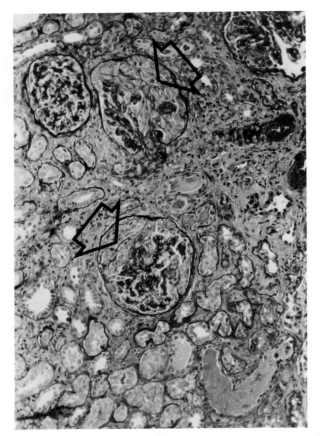

Figure 9-20. Crescentic glomerulonephritis. Two glomeruli have proliferative crescents (arrows). Note tubular casts and interstitial inflammation. (Hematoxylin and eosin ×120)

whereas *small vessel vasculitis* involves smaller vessels. *Wegener's granulomatosis* is a granulomatous vasculitis. The clinical setting will vary with the disease, but in general adults are more frequently affected than children. Systemic symptoms are common, with many organ systems involved in addition to the kidneys. The respiratory tract and kidneys are extensively involved in Wegener's granulomatosis. Laboratory studies will usually reveal a leukocytosis, eosinophilia, and an elevated sedimentation rate. The renal lesion is manifested by hematuria and commonly renal failure. The prognosis is poor without treatment. Wegener's granulomatosis is best treated with cyclophosphamide and other vasculitis by corticosteroids.

Pathogenesis and Histology
Vasculitis is believed to be an immune-complex disease, but this hypothesis is not proven in all cases. Large and medium-sized vessels are involved in

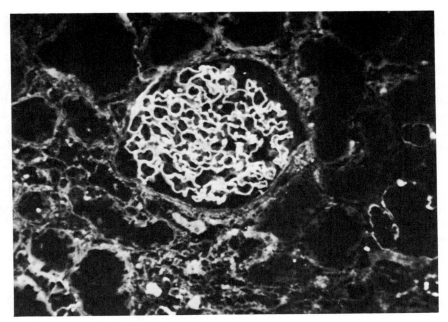

Figure 9-21. Immunofluorescence microscopy demonstrating linear glomerular fluorescence of IgG typical of anti-GBM antibody.

polyarteritis nodosa with a polymorphonuclear infiltrate throughout the vessel wall. Smaller vessels are involved in *microscopic vasculitis*. Giant cells are present in vessel walls in Wegener's granulomatosis. Glomerular lesions are usually focal and proliferative. Areas of necrosis or crescent formation are seen at times.

Hemolytic Uremic Syndrome (HUS) and Thrombotic Thrombocytopenic Purpura (TTP)

HUS and TTP are vascular diseases that have a similar clinical and pathologic picture. HUS commonly involves infants and young children, while TTP affects adults. A hemolytic anemia with distorted "helmet-shaped" red blood cells is common to both diseases. This anemia has been called *microangiopathic* and is felt to be caused by intravascular fibrin deposition. A decreased number of circulating platelets (thrombocytopenia) is also found in both, as are hematuria and renal failure. In HUS the renal failure is abrupt, but the outlook for reversal and long-term preservation of adequate renal function is fairly good if the patient lives. In TTP the renal failure develops more insidiously, but the prognosis for survival and recovery of kidney function is poor. Fever and jaundice as well as transient neurologic signs are seen in TTP, while gastrointestinal bleeding is more common in HUS. Serum complement levels are normal or slightly depressed. Antiplatelet agents and plasmapheresis hold promise for the future as methods of treatment which are at least partially effective for both diseases.

Pathogenesis and Histology

The pathogenesis is unknown, but intravascular deposition of fibrin and platelet thrombi is felt to be responsible for the vascular injury as well as the hemolytic anemia. The lesions frequently seen in the renal arterioles consist of fibrinoid necrosis and intimal swelling with intraluminal thrombi. Vascular lesions in HUS may be so severe as to cause both tubular and glomerular (cortical) necrosis. Glomerular lesions by light microscopy range from focal necrosis with intracapillary thrombi to occasional proliferative crescent formation. Immunofluorescent techniques will reveal vascular and glomerular fibrin but no immunoglobulins. Capillary basement membranes are thickened with finely granular subendothelial deposits, and fibrin and platelets may be identified by electron microscopy.

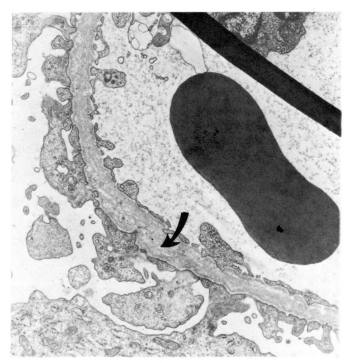

Figure 9-22. Electron micrograph of a glomerular capillary basement membrane in Alport's syndrome. The basement membrane appears "moth eaten" because of intermittent lucent areas (arrow). This finding is typical of but not limited to Alport's syndrome.

Hereditary Glomerulonephritis

(Synonym: Alport's syndrome)

Hereditary nephritis occurs in families, but the exact mode of genetic transmission is unknown. An autosomal dominant inheritance is most commonly suggested. Males are involved more frequently and with more severe disease than females. Deafness and ocular abnormalities are often present. The most prevalent renal manifestation of the disease is hematuria with progression to renal failure in males, but significant proteinuria may also occur.

The pathogenesis is unknown, and the glomerular alterations by light microscopy are nondescript. Interstitial cells containing cholesterol are commonly noted, and these "foam cells" are characteristic of the disease. Immunofluorescence studies are negative, but thinning, splitting and a moth-eaten appearance of the glomerular capillary basement membrane is noted on electron microscopy (Fig. 9-22).

BIBLIOGRAPHY

R. J. Glassock. The nephrotic syndrome. *Hosp. Prac.* 14: 105–129, November 1979.

R. J. Glassock, A. H. Cohen, C. M. Bennett, et al: Primary glomerular diseases. In *The Kidney*, 2nd ed., B. M. Brenner and F. C. Rector, Jr. (Eds.). Philadelphia: W. B. Saunders, 1981, pp. 1351–1492.

Glomerular diseases (by numerous authors). In *Pediatric Kidney Disease*, C. M. Edelmann, Jr., (Ed.). Boston: Little, Brown, 1978, pp. 586–723.

M. Kashgarian, J. P. Hayslett, and B. H. Spargo. Renal disease. *Am. J. Pathol.* 89: 187–272, 1977.

Primary glomerulopathies (by numerous authors). In *Strauss and Welt's Diseases of the Kidney*, 3rd ed., L. E. Earley and C. W. Gottschalk (Eds.). Boston: Little, Brown, 1979, pp. 541–813.
  Includes discussion of clinical aspects of glomerulonephritis and nephrotic syndrome, pathology and immunopathology.

C. B. Wilson and F. J. Dixon. Immunologic mechanisms in nephritogenesis. *Hosp. Prac.* 14: 57–69, April 1979.

10
Congenital, Hereditary, and Interstitial Renal Disease

Congenital, hereditary, and interstitial diseases are responsible for roughly half of the incidence of end-stage renal failure. A complete list of all the known conditions in this category would include numerous esoteric diseases, rarely seen even by specialists and almost never by the average physician. In this chapter we shall focus instead on the relatively few problems that are the most frequent troublemakers.

CONGENITAL DISEASES

Congenital diseases are present at birth but are usually not genetically inherited.

Agenesis (complete absence) of one kidney occurs in about one out of 1500 people. This fact is worth remembering, because the assumption that everyone has two kidneys occasionally has led to the surgical removal of a solitary kidney—not a wise thing to do. Before any manipulation is performed on one kidney, it is prudent to be sure the patient has another one.

Hypoplastic kidneys are small, otherwise relatively normal kidneys. They are small because of either a decreased number of nephrons or the diminished size of individual nephrons. Hypoplastic kidneys can be unilateral or bilateral. The function of these kidneys may be impaired enough to cause renal failure if both kidneys are hypoplastic; it is estimated that about 20% of renal failure in childhood may be attributable to bilateral hypoplastic kidneys. On the other hand, the presence of one hypoplastic kidney usually does not result in abnormal renal function or produce symptoms. Statistics based on autopsies indicate that the incidence of this condition in adults is about one in 500.

Unilateral hypoplasia, like agenesis, assumes importance when a patient has a problem requiring medical evaluation or intervention. If intravenous pyelography is performed, the discovery of a small kidney may lead to a diagnosis of unilateral hypoplasia. It is important to remember that a diminution of kidney size may also be caused by conditions such as renal artery stenosis, vascular disease in the kidney, vesicoureteral reflux, or severe infection. The cortical scars and corresponding radiographic defects that may result from these diseases help to distinguish them from hypoplasia, in which the kidney usually has a normal contour.

Renal dysplasia results from an abnormal development of the kidney. In contrast to hypoplastic kidneys where things are fairly normal except for the number or size of functioning nephron units, dysplastic kidneys have a confused anatomic organization. Things just haven't been put together right, and elements of nonrenal tissue, including cartilage, may be present. Dysplastic kidneys actually represent a group of malformations that may be solid or cystic, large or small, with variable functional derangement. The medulla is usually undersized, and glomeruli remain small and immature. There is frequent association between renal dysplasia and abnormalities of the ureter, bladder, and urethra. In many instances these abnormalities have produced an obstruction to urine flow that may have played a role in producing dysplasia. The presence of two dysplastic kidneys can result in uremia, and in children this is a fairly common cause of renal failure, usually noted in the setting of an obstructed or abnormal lower urinary tract.

HEREDITARY RENAL DISEASES

Hereditary kidney diseases are passed on from generation to generation via genetic mechanisms. Not all of these inherited disorders lead to renal insufficiency, but those that do may account for up to 10% of all cases of end-stage renal failure.

Polycystic Renal Disease

Cysts in the kidneys have many causes. For instance, they may be present in dysplastic kidneys. Solitary cysts that are usually not inherited may occur in otherwise normal kidneys; typically they cause no symptoms or problems. Hereditary polycystic disease is usually not benign, however, because the cysts tend to enlarge, squeezing and disrupting normal renal tissue as they expand. Renal failure usually ensues.

There are two principal types of hereditary polycystic kidneys:

1. *Infantile polycystic kidneys,* inherited as an autosomal recessive trait, are usually enlarged at birth with dilated cystic collecting ducts. Renal function is usually insufficient to support life to adulthood. Infantile polycystic kidneys are frequently associated with hepatic fibrosis, which occasionally produces portal hypertension.

2. *Adult polycystic kidneys,* inherited as an autosomal dominant trait, also enlarge and are associated with renal failure. Decline in renal function is

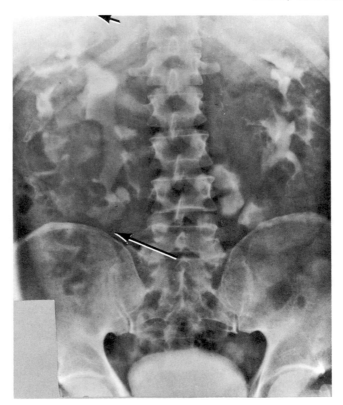

Figure 10-1. Intravenous pyelogram of a patient with adult polycystic kidney disease. The arrows outline the large size of the right kidney. The usual calyceal pattern is disrupted by cysts.

slow, however, and most patients are in their forties or older before renal failure is present. About 7% of patients with end-stage renal disease have adult polycystic kidneys. Pain or hematuria from bleeding cysts as well as hypertension may be noted in these patients. Figure 10-1 shows how large the kidneys can be and how the pelvis and calyces can be distorted by the cysts.

Hereditary Nephritis (Alport's syndrome)

This disorder is discussed in the chapter on Glomerulopathies.

Medullary Cystic Disease

As the name implies, small medullary cysts are found in this condition. Unlike polycystic disease, however, it is associated with small kidneys. Unfortunately, this disease also leads to renal failure, which often occurs in early adulthood.

The name *familial juvenile nephronophthisis* has been applied to a very similar entity, also associated with medullary cysts, which causes renal failure in childhood or adolescence. It has been argued, in fact, that these are the same disease, differing only in the age at which they cause renal failure. Familial juvenile nephronophthisis is inherited as an autosomal recessive trait, however, whereas medullary cystic disease has an autosomal dominant genetic transmission. Clinical features that are similar include polyuria, polydypsia, anemia, and an unremarkable urinary sediment. Impaired renal ability to conserve sodium is a common finding, often associated with an impressive intake of salt.

Metabolic Defects Causing Renal Disease

In previous chapters we referred to some metabolic defects, a number of them inherited, that interfere with certain aspects of renal function but do not usually cause renal damage or failure. Renal glucosuria and diabetes insipidus are examples of such disorders. There are other hereditary biochemical defects that cause the abnormal accumulation of metabolic products within kidney parenchyma, leading eventually to kidney failure. Several diseases in the latter category merit brief mention here, though they are quite uncommon.

There are two different hereditary disorders leading to *oxalosis,* an accumulation of oxalate in the kidney that eventually leads to renal failure. Unfortunately, the oxalate also causes severe damage to other tissues and becomes deposited in transplanted kidneys, so the benefits of renal transplantation are limited and temporary.

Cystine is deposited in kidney parenchyma in patients with *cystinosis,* an autosomal recessive defect in cystine metabolism. The cystine accumulation leads to renal tubular defects producing glucosuria as well as increased urinary excretion of uric acid, amino acids, phosphate, and bicarbonate (Fanconi's syndrome). Increased cystine deposition eventually produces renal failure.

Fabry's disease is an X-linked recessive defect in 2-galactosidase activity leading an accumulation of glycosphingolipid in glomeruli. Renal failure can occur but is not the rule.

Other Hereditary Disorders

There are a number of rather rare hereditary conditions that may affect the kidneys but do not fall into any of the preceding categories. An example of these is the *nail-patella syndrome,* a condition characterized by dystrophic fingernails, malformations of the radius, and absent or hypoplastic patellae. Thirty to 40% of those with this syndrome have renal disease manifest by proteinuria and, rarely, renal failure. The characteristic pathologic abnormality is a lucent area in the glomerular basement membrane. This disease is inherited in an autosomal dominant pattern.

Another unusual disorder, *familial recurrent hematuria,* is associated with a very thin glomerular basement membrane and usually normal renal function. The glomerular findings and the fact that this is a familial problem serve to distinguish it from the two types of recurrent hematuria described in the previous chapter.

INTERSTITIAL NEPHRITIS

Surrounding and interspersed among the glomeruli, tubules, ducts and blood vessels of the kidney is a tissue space known as the renal *interstitium;* it contains connective-tissue cells, fibrils, extracellular fluid, and some other cells whose role is not clear. In the normal kidney the renal tubules and vessels are closely fitted next to each other, and the interstitium makes up only a small portion of the kidney tissue. When there is inflammation of the interstitium, however, there is a clear separation of renal tubules from each other by edema or fibrosis and usually an infiltration of acute or chronic inflammatory cells. Such a process may occur as a part of glomerular, vascular, congenital, or hereditary diseases. In some cases, however, none of these other conditions appear to be present, and interstitial inflammation is the most conspicuous finding on microscopic examination of renal tissue. The picture is then called *acute interstitial nephritis* or *chronic interstitial nephritis;* these two categories are usually separable on the basis of their different clinical presentations, histopathology and pathogenesis.

Acute Interstitial Nephritis

Except for acute allograft rejection (see Chapter 14), most episodes of acute interstitial nephritis are associated with the administration of drugs. Penicillin, methicillin, ampicillin, diuretics, rifampin, anticonvulsants, phenindione, and allopurinol all have been associated with acute interstitial nephritis. The common presentation is one of fever, skin rash, and hematuria with a variable but generally reversible decrease in renal function. Eosinophils are present in the urinary sediment and in increased numbers in the peripheral blood. A biopsy of renal tissue will show edema of the interstitium, frequently with infiltration by polymorphonuclear cells and eosinophils. Red blood cells may be seen in the tubules, which are surrounded by inflammatory cells.

Perhaps the most important thing to remember is that drugs can cause acute interstitial nephritis. In medical practice today the administration of drugs is so commonplace that we may overlook their possible role in a patient with unexplained fever, skin rash, or hematuria. When the relationship is suspect, administration of drugs that might be responsible should cease, because continued use may possibly lead to irreversible renal failure.

The pathogenesis of drug-related acute interstitial nephritis would seem to involve the immune system, although for the most part this is unproven. Antibodies against tubular basement membrane have been described in patients with methicillin-induced nephritis, but their presence alone does not prove that they caused the disease. Further investigation will be needed to reveal the exact mechanisms that produce acute interstitial nephritis.

Chronic Interstitial Nephritis

Chronic interstitial nephritis represents a diagnostic challenge to physicians akin to those that confronted Sherlock Holmes. Unlike glomerular disease, where proteinuria or hematuria may lead to the detection of the problem at an early stage, chronic interstitial nephritis is not usually associated with significant urinary abnormalities. Unfortunately, this means that most patients come to their doctors with fairly advanced kidney failure. In any patient with renal insufficiency of unknown etiology, the possibility of chronic interstitial nephritis should be suspected and investigated. The reward could be the discovery of an offending agent whose removal will lead to stabilization or even improvement in renal function.

The kidneys are often small in patients with chronic interstitial nephritis. Lymphocytes, plasma cells, and other mononuclear cells may be seen in the interstitium, where fibrous tissue has replaced tubules that have been destroyed (Fig. 10-2). Other tubules are atrophied or dilated and filled with casts.

Chronic interstitial nephritis may evolve from a variety of different insults to the kidney. For instance, irradiation of the kidneys has been responsible for some cases, mainly by producing arteriolar hyperplasia and ischemia. (It is now common practice to shield the kidneys during therapeutic irradiation treatments in order to prevent this complication.) Chronic hypertension may have similar consequences. Prolonged exposure to heavy metals such as lead and cadmium has also been associated with chronic tubulointerstitial changes, although this is an uncommon cause of end-stage renal disease.

Mechanical factors that interfere with the normal drainage of urine from the kidneys are fairly common causes of chronic interstitial nephritis. Among the most important of these are urinary tract obstruction and vesicoureteral reflux. Obstruction may be caused by various lesions and is quite common in older men with hypertrophy of the prostate gland. Reflux of urine from the bladder up the ureter during micturition is not unusual in newborns, but it usually disappears during early childhood. When it persists, it can lead to progressive renal disease. Though vesicoureteral reflux can be corrected surgically, such treatment may be futile if renal function is already decreased.

In the past, bacterial infection was considered one of the most frequent causes of chronic interstitial nephritis. This misconception developed in part from the fact that chronic vesicoureteral reflux, urinary tract obstruction, analgesic nephropathy, and nephrolithiasis are all commonly associated with infection as well as with interstitial nephritis. The renal lesions seen in these conditions were blamed on infection and described as examples of *pyelonephritis*. Thus most articles on "chronic pyelonephritis" written in past decades

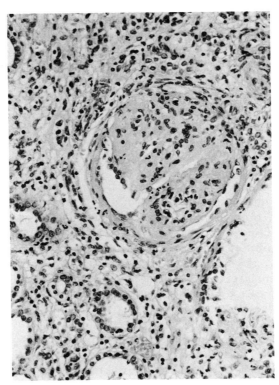

Figure 10-2. Renal biopsy specimen from a patient with chronic interstitial nephritis secondary to vesicoureteral reflux. The glomerulus is sclerotic, and the tubules are separated by mononuclear cells and fibrosis. (Hematoxylin and eosin ×150)

included many cases of chronic interstitial nephritis that we would now attribute to other primary causes. We realize now that chronic infection without urinary tract abnormalities rarely leads to renal failure, though it is possible that secondary infection may accelerate the disease process that some other condition has initiated.

Not all chronic tubulointerstitial diseases have an obvious cause. Residents of the Danube River valley in Yugoslavia, Rumania, and Bulgaria, for instance, are at risk for development of interstitial nephritis if they reside for over 10 years in this area. Despite intensive detective work, no etiologic agent can yet be incriminated, although the specific localization obviously favors an environmental agent.

Analgesic nephropathy deserves special mention because it is responsible for a large fraction of end-stage renal disease in some countries and may be more prevalent than we realize in others, including the United States. This is a chronic interstitial nephritis occurring in people who continually take analgesic mixtures for many years. Since the first description of this condition, it was assumed to be related to prolonged use of phenacetin, but in more recent years, while the entity of analgesic nephropathy is unquestioned, the nature of the exact offending agent remains a controversial issue. In the past, most combinations of pain-relieving drugs contained phenacetin, which is metabolized to n-acetyl-p-aminophenol (acetaminophen), but aspirin and caffeine were also common components. Controversy arises from the fact that it has been difficult to produce interstitial nephritis in animals fed phenacetin. However, since renal lesions are rare in patients with rheumatoid arthritis who ingest large amounts of aspirin, it seems unlikely that aspirin alone produces chronic renal failure. It is possible that a combination of analgesic agents is necessary to produce the lesions.

Although the exact agent causing renal damage is unclear, the clinical setting is quite consistent. Patients have usually ingested large amounts of analgesic agents containing phenacetin for at least 15 years. Females predominate, and a family history of analgesic overuse is common. Patients have an elderly appearance, a high incidence of peptic ulcers, may have renal papillary necrosis, and eventually develop kidney failure. The most important aspect of treatment is to stop the use of analgesics, which will usually arrest the progression of disease if late-stage renal damage is not already present. The diagnosis of analgesic-abuse nephropathy is very difficult to make because patients usually do not consider over-the-counter medicines as "drugs." They may also deny that they take analgesics and may continue to use them in spite of contrary advice from their physicians. Persistent questioning of patients and family members regarding analgesic use may be rewarding if the cause of renal insufficiency is unknown.

In summary, even though chronic intestitial nephritis is difficult to detect early, a careful search for a specific cause is worthwhile, since many patients may benefit from removal of an offending agent or correction of an anatomic abnormality.

BIBLIOGRAPHY

R. H. Heptinstall. Interstitial nephritis. In *Pathology of the Kidney*, 2nd ed. Boston: Little, Brown, 1974, pp. 821–836.

A. Spitzer, J. Bernstein, J. Kissane, and K. Gardner, Jr. Neonatal, congenital and hereditary disorders. In *Pediatric Kidney Disease*, C. M. Edelmann, Jr. (Ed.). Boston: Little, Brown, 1978, pp. 537–586.

W. Suki and G. Eknoyan. Tubulo-interstitial disease. In *The Kidney*, B. M. Brenner and F. C. Rector, Jr. (Eds.). Philadelphia: W. B. Saunders, 1976, pp. 1113–1144.

11
Acute Renal Failure

England was a dangerous place in 1941. Adolph Hitler ruled most of the European continent, and a landing on the British Isles by his forces was considered imminent. In an apparent effort to pave the way for such an invasion, German bombers flew nightly missions over London and other English cities, dropping tons of explosives. Casualties on the ground were high. Hospitals were crowded with severely injured people, some of whom had been crushed in the rubble of collapsing buildings.

This grim, chaotic scene was the setting for an important medical observation made by Bywaters and his colleagues. After successful treatment of major injuries and apparent recovery from shock, some patients were found to be producing virtually no urine. As more days passed without significant urine output, these patients began to show the signs of kidney failure, such as puffiness, pulmonary congestion, nausea, and vomiting. Blood urea concentration became grossly elevated, and serum potassium rose to dangerous levels. Death from renal failure seemed only a short time away. But then, a week or 10 days after the injury, a small increase in urine volume might be observed, followed by a further increase the next day. Additional improvement in urine output would be seen on succeeding days, followed by a reduction in serum levels of urea and potassium. A week after the first indication of recovery the urine volume might be normal or even excessive, though blood chemistry values were still grossly abnormal. During this phase of recovery the patient might still succumb to electrolyte disturbances because the damaged kidneys were as yet unable to regulate the excretion of sodium and potassium. If he got past this danger period, however, renal function would be back to normal within a month or two.

Others died before any improvement of kidney function occurred. Many suffered intractable cardiac arrhythmias, which appeared as serum potassium concentrations rose relentlessly to high levels. Some, uremic and debilitated, succumbed to infection. At autopsy, most of these patients had no gross anatomical disruption of the urinary tract, though their kidneys were pale and swollen. Under the microscope the glomeruli appeared normal, but large areas could be seen where the tubular cells were necrotic and the tubular lumina were filled with their debris.

Table 11-1. Some Clinical Situations Associated with Acute Renal Tubular Necrosis

Problems characterized by renal ischemia
  Shock—due to hemorrhage or drastic loss of extracellular fluid
        —due to severe cardiac insufficiency (cardiogenic shock)
    Major vascular surgery—especially aortic surgery, often involving major blood loss,
      hypotension and cross-clamping of the aorta
Problems caused by nephrotoxic substances
  Transfusion reactions (products of hemolysis)
  Muscle breakdown without severe injury (products of myolysis)
  Toxicity due to antibiotics, especially aminoglycosides and some cephalosporins
  Toxicity from radiographic contrast agents
  Poisoning with mercury or other heavy metals, carbon tetrachloride, ethylene gly-
    col, methanol, others.
Problems involving both ischemia and nephrotoxic substances
  Septic shock (endotoxin)
  Severe injury—especially crush injuries and burns (tissue breakdown products and
    shock)
  Septic abortion (blood loss and toxic bacterial products)

This type of sudden renal failure is still very much with us. In fact, it was with us long before World War II, though not on such a large scale, and the sporadic case reports had been largely overlooked. After Bywaters and his associates brought this problem to the attention of the medical world, it became apparent that acute kidney failure might occur in many settings. The most common of these are listed in Table 11-1. As indicated in the table, these situations are characterized by renal ischemia, the presence of nephrotoxic substances, or a combination of both.

In all these circumstances a similar picture may be seen. A major insult is followed immediately or within hours by abrupt and almost total failure of kidney function. Usually the problem becomes obvious because of severe oliguria (a drastically reduced urine flow often less than 100 ml/day). In a few cases the patient continues to produce a normal volume of urine that is obviously of poor quality, since clearance measurements and other tests reflect an almost total loss of the excretory and regulatory functions of the kidney. Examination of kidney tissue obtained by biopsy or at autopsy shows the same patchy tubular necrosis that was observed in the victims of the London air raids. If the patient survives long enough, recovery of renal function occurs in a matter of weeks, usually heralded by increasing urine volume. Progressive improvement of glomerular filtration follows, with complete recovery of the regulatory functions of the tubules sometimes taking a bit longer. In a typical case urine volume begins to increase one to two weeks following the acute loss of function, often on or around the tenth day, and normal function is restored after a month or two. Occasionally, severe renal failure has persisted for a month or more—a situation that raises doubts about eventual recovery and forces consideration of other possible causes of the failure.

The syndrome we have just described has a confusing number of names. Early investigators called it *acute tubular necrosis,* reflecting the most striking abnormality in the kidney tissues as well as their belief that necrosis of the tubules was responsible for the renal failure. Some later workers, whose experiments will be described shortly, suggested that the term *vasomotor nephropathy* would be more in keeping with what they considered the true cause of the disorder. For a while, this was the "in" terminology. The fence-straddlers, who wanted to describe the syndrome without taking a position about its pathogenesis, often chose the designation *acute renal failure.* Acute renal failure is certainly descriptive of the problem—no one can argue with that— but unfortunately it also describes a number of other conditions in which an abrupt cessation of kidney function occurs. Thus this term is not specific.

We will use the term *acute tubular necrosis* for the syndrome that has been described. This decision is rather arbitrary, and you should be aware that those who refer to vasomotor nephropathy are talking about exactly the same problem. Some of those who speak of acute renal failure mean the same thing, too, but we shall use acute renal failure to refer to a larger group of disorders that includes acute tubular necrosis.

PATHOGENESIS OF ACUTE TUBULAR NECROSIS

Despite extensive investigations by many workers, there is still no consensus about the mechanisms that cause renal failure in acute tubular necrosis. A number of different explanations can claim impressive experimental support. We shall summarize the major theories and the evidence for them.

Tubular Obstruction

The early students of acute tubular necrosis saw the morphological changes we have described—necrotic tubular cells that had sloughed into the tubular lumina—and had no difficulty explaining the oliguria and renal failure: The plumbing was clogged with debris. It was indeed noted that the cellular necrosis was only patchy, with areas of normal-appearing tubular cells interspersed among the dead ones; but it seemed reasonable to believe that a tubule that appeared normal on one microscopic section might be severely damaged at some other point. This might explain why the ostensibly normal tubules were not producing urine. It was also suggested that since these kidneys were swollen, any tubules that had not been damaged might still be closed off by increased pressure within the kidney.

Back-Leak

Another hypothesis suggested that the injured tubules had lost their capacity for discriminating resorption. According to this view, virtually all the glomerular filtrate was diffusing passively through the damaged cells into the peritubular circulation, leaving essentially none to form urine.

Vasomotor Factors

In the 1960s Oken and his associates proposed a different concept about the pathogenesis of renal failure in acute tubular necrosis. Their experiments utilized animals in which renal damage was produced by methods such as injecting glycerol intramuscularly or giving uranyl nitrate. The kidneys were studied by micropuncture before and immediately following the administration of these nephrotoxic insults.

These investigators reasoned that if tubular blockage is a mechanism of renal failure, hydrostatic pressure within the lumina of the proximal tubules near the glomeruli should rise as obstruction is developing downstream. Instead, they found that intraluminal pressure falls markedly and rapidly at the onset of renal injury. Oken and his co-workers reasoned that this must reflect a sharp decrease in glomerular filtration and that this decrease, rather than tubular obstruction, was the primary event in the rapidly developing renal failure. The decreased glomerular filtration was presumed to result from a fall of hydrostatic pressure in the glomeruli, caused in turn by changes in the muscular tone of the afferent or efferent arterioles or both. These investigators suggested, therefore, that the term *vasomotor-nephropathy* would be more physiologically appropriate for this disorder than acute tubular necrosis, which was now believed to be a secondary development.

The vasomotor theory received further support from experiments in other laboratories which showed a relationship between the amount of renin in the kidneys of an experimental animal and the susceptibility of those kidneys to acute tubular necrosis. You will recall that renin is found in the arteriolar walls of the juxtaglomerular apparatus, where it may regulate vascular tone by promoting formation of angiotensin, a potent vasoconstrictor. So it might be expected that a reduction of the amount of renin available would reduce the potential for arteriolar constriction. Maneuvers such as prolonged sodium or potassium loading, which reduce the amount of renin in the kidneys, also protect against experimentally induced acute renal failure, supporting the argument that acute tubular necrosis is caused by vasoconstriction. It must be pointed out, however, that some experimental evidence does not support a relationship between renin and acute tubular necrosis.

An interesting variation of the vasomotor theory has been proposed by Thurau and Boylan. They suggest that oliguria in acute tubular necrosis results from the inability of damaged proximal tubules to perform their normal resorptive functions. This breakdown causes a momentary surge of unreabsorbed sodium and chloride to be delivered to the juxtaglomerular apparatus, where normal feedback mechanisms operate via renin and arteriolar constriction to produce a drastic reduction in glomerular filtration. This virtual shutdown of filtration, which persists until the tubules have recovered their resorptive capacities, can thus be regarded as a mechanism that protects the body against catastrophic losses of sodium and chloride. From this perspective, Thurau and Boylan suggest that the resulting clinical picture should really be called "acute renal success"!

Changes in Glomerular Capillaries

If a decrease of glomerular filtration rate is an important early event in the oliguria of acute tubular necrosis and not just the consequence of tubular blockage, why does it occur? There appear to be two possibilities: Either the hydrostatic pressure within the glomerular capillaries is reduced or the permeability of the capillaries themselves is impaired. Oken and his co-workers, who popularized the vasomotor theory, focused on hydrostatic pressure and considered permeability changes unlikely, since the glomeruli in acute tubular necrosis appear normal under the microscope.

Recently, however, some studies have suggested that the ultrafiltration coefficient of the glomeruli (K_F, a measure of glomerular permeability) is reduced in at least some forms of experimental acute tubular necrosis. It is possible that these results reflect only an acute decrease in glomerular filtering area because of decreased hydrostatic pressure and consequent capillary shrinkage. On the other hand, there might be a change in the characteristics of the capillary wall. The latter possibility is favored by the finding on electron microscopy of fused foot processes and other structural changes in the glomerular epithelial cells in some experiments. So it is conceivable that injury to the epithelial cells or other parts of the glomerular barrier might result in a marked reduction of filtration.

Perspective

Since the description of acute tubular necrosis in 1941, we have seen the rise and fall of at least two widely accepted explanations for its oliguria and renal failure. The theory of tubular obstruction (possibly combined with abnormal back-leak) held sway for many years until the general acceptance of the vasomotor theory. In recent years, however, tubular obstruction has been resurrected as a factor of pathogenetic importance, supported by work from a number of laboratories. And other explanations, such as those involving ultrastructural changes in the glomeruli, are also emerging. The controversy is likely to be with us for some time to come.

DIAGNOSTIC CONSIDERATIONS IN ACUTE RENAL FAILURE

Any abrupt and essentially total failure of renal function may be termed acute renal failure. The clinical-pathological syndrome we have described as acute tubular necrosis (alias vasomotor nephropathy) is an important cause of

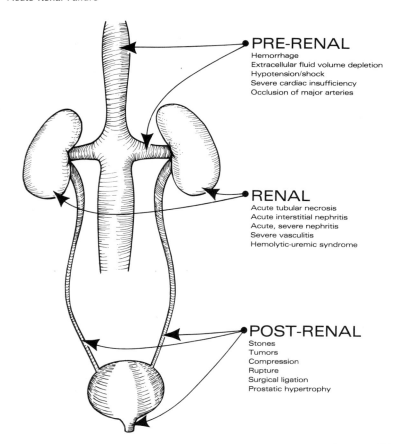

Figure 11-1. General areas and specific disorders to be considered as possible causes of acute renal failure.

acute renal failure, but not the only cause. Since many of the other conditions causing acute renal failure call for treatment that is very different from the treatment of acute tubular necrosis, it is most important to distinguish between them. Such discrimination may be difficult, since many of these problems have clinical features very similar to those of acute tubular necrosis, including severe oliguria or anuria.

The conditions that cause acute renal failure can be classified as postrenal, intrinsic renal, or prerenal (Fig. 11-1).

Postrenal Difficulties—Failures in the Plumbing

Postrenal disorders include any problem that causes renal failure by interfering with the flow of urine from the kidneys to the exterior of the body. Such interference may result from obstruction or disruption of the urinary tract.

An obstruction that blocks the flow of urine may occur at any level from the renal pelvis to the urethra. The ureter may be obstructed by a tumor of the renal pelvis or the ureter itself, or the flow of urine into the bladder may be shut off by carcinoma of the bladder. A strategically placed stone may accomplish the same mischief. Ureters may also be compressed shut from the outside by tumors, retroperitoneal fibrosis, or aneurysms, and occasionally a ureter has been litigated mistakenly during pelvic surgery.

Urine that has reached the bladder may be prevented from leaving by bladder dysfunction, a bladder stone (rare in the United States), or an enlargement of the prostate gland in males. The last condition is rather common in older men.

Disruption of the ureters or bladder may result from trauma or surgery. When this occurs, urine leaks from the collecting system into the retroperitoneal space or pelvis, where it is reabsorbed and recycled by the kidneys. Though the kidneys are working overtime, no urine appears on the outside, and the patient grows progressively more azotemic.

Since a normal person has two kidneys, obstruction or disruption of a single ureter will not cause oliguria or renal failure. The remaining kidney, if normal, can carry on splendidly—so well, in fact, that the loss of one kidney may pass without notice. Both ureters must be blocked or ruptured in order to cause acute renal failure, and this requirement reduces the chances that the trouble is at the ureteral level. That is not much comfort to the physician trying to unravel the problem, however. There is a significant number of people walking around with only one functioning kidney because they were born that way or because one kidney is already out of order due to obstruction, infarction, or the like. Many of them don't know that they are living with one kidney. Under such circumstances, it only takes obstruction of one ureter to precipitate disaster. Therefore, interruption of the collecting system at any level must be considered in the patient who has acute renal failure.

The patient's history and findings usually provide clues that can make it likely or unlikely that acute renal failure is due to a postrenal cause. Rupture of the bladder or ureter is unlikely in the absence of severe trauma. A past history of renal stones or tumors in the urinary tract increases the chances of obstruction due to these causes. Movement of a stone into a ureter usually causes severe and characteristic pain. Oliguria that occurs immediately after surgery, especially a hysterectomy, forces consideration of a possible surgical accident, though well-trained gynecologists are alert to this hazard and avoid the ureters scrupulously. Prostatic hypertrophy is almost exclusively a disease of older men, and the patient, who may have had difficulties voiding for a long time, is likely to be painfully aware of his distended bladder if he is alert. Other clinical circumstances, such as a recent episode of shock, may point strongly away from postrenal causes and toward acute tubular necrosis.

Armed with the available information in each case, the physician must decide whether obstruction or disruption of the urinary tract can be excluded beyond a reasonable doubt as the cause of the patient's renal failure or whether further studies are necessary. A wrong judgment here can be very serious, since the problems that cause postrenal failure call for surgical intervention in many cases and are not likely to improve spontaneously. Additional information is often necessary to exclude such conditions with confidence.

Excretory urography (intravenous pyelography), which is the primary method for examining the urinary tract under most circumstances, is often unsatisfactory in acute renal failure because the kidneys do not process the contrast agent well enough to show the structures. In some centers, high doses of contrast material are used in combination with tomography of the kidneys; it is claimed that enough information can be obtained by this technique to exclude urinary tract obstruction. If not, it is often necessary to resort to retrograde pyelography—an invasive procedure one is reluctant to undertake in a person who is quite ill, as these patients usually are. A unilateral retrograde study is sufficient, since demonstration of a patent and intact urinary tract up to one normal-appearing kidney excludes obstruction as a cause of acute renal failure. Noninvasive ultrasonography of the kidneys, which is becoming increasingly sophisticated, may soon make retrograde pyelography unnecessary in most cases. If it can be demonstrated with confidence by this technique that there is no hydronephrosis (distention of the renal pelvis with fluid), obstruction to the outflow of urine is highly unlikely as a cause of renal failure.

Intrinsic Renal Failure

By far the most common cause of acute renal failure that is intrinsic to the kidney itself is acute tubular necrosis. On rare occasions a process within the glomeruli or small vessels of the kidney, such as acute poststreptococcal glomerulonephritis, vascular inflammation or the hemolytic-uremic syndrome, may cause confusion. These diseases may be sufficiently severe to cause a sudden reduction of renal function with oliguria so striking that the picture can be mistaken for acute tubular necrosis. Usually the circumstances, such as the sudden appearance of hematuria and red cell casts in a child who was otherwise well after a recent streptococcal infection, will arouse suspicion that the problem is not acute tubular necrosis. If there is real doubt about the diagnosis, a renal biopsy can resolve the question, though this is rarely necessary.

Acute interstitial nephritis (described in Chapter 10) has clinical features very like those of acute tubular necrosis and is treated in much the same way. There are some significant differences, however. Acute interstitial nephritis is a hypersensitivity reaction that involves the kidneys, so renal biopsy will show inflammatory cells in the interstitium rather than tubular necrosis, and eosinophils are sometimes found in the urine. Recovery from acute interstitial nephritis usually begins when (and not before) the agent that caused the reaction is removed, so identification and withdrawal of drugs that may be responsible is most important. Steroid hormones may accelerate this recovery, but they are useless and potentially harmful in acute tubular necrosis.

Prerenal Causes of Acute Failure

Failure of the circulatory system to supply the kidneys with a large enough blood flow under adequate pressure may result in acute renal failure, even though the kidneys themselves may be perfectly normal. Such failure is described as prerenal, and the kidneys are said to be *underperfused* or *hypoperfused*.

Prerenal failure is usually associated with markedly decreased cardiac output, often caused by a major loss of blood or extracellular fluid volume. The patient may be in clinical shock, in which case the renal dysfunction comes as no surprise. In more subtle circumstances the serious depletion of circulating volume may not be obvious, and the patient may even have normal blood pressure while lying flat in bed, though it may plunge alarmingly if he stands up. Under such circumstances the kidneys may be among the organs whose circulation is being curtailed in an apparent attempt to maintain blood flow to the heart, lungs, and brain, and renal failure may be the alarm that brings the poor state of the circulation to clinical attention.

Very severe heart failure may occasionally cause the picture of acute renal failure due to hypoperfusion. This is in contrast to milder degrees of cardiac insufficiency, where usually the only obvious renal manifestation is a tendency to retain sodium.

A sudden mechanical interruption of renal blood flow, such as embolization to the renal arteries, also may be responsible for acute renal failure, though this is rare.

The Usual Dilemma

Sometimes, it is fairly easy to identify the cause of a patient's acute renal failure. The clinical setting may point clearly to an obstructive problem, which can then be demonstrated unequivocally. In certain circumstances we may be virtually certain that the patient has acute tubular necrosis or that renal perfusion is so poor that glomerular filtration is not taking place.

In other situations, however, it is very difficult to be certain about the cause of renal failure. The usual problem is one of trying to decide whether the immediate cause of the patient's renal failure is hypoperfusion or acute tubular necrosis. Hypoperfusion is obviously a circulatory problem, but acute tubular necrosis is often associated with circulatory problems also.

Let's consider an example: An elderly man has a history of hypertension and moderate cardiac insufficiency, for which he has been under treatment. One afternoon he notices abdominal pain, which becomes more severe over the course of several hours. When he gets up to walk to the bathroom, he collapses and is then brought to the hospital. In the emergency room he is found to be hypotensive. After hurried evaluation and consultation, he is taken to the operating room, where a leaking aortic aneurysm is found with over 2 liters of blood in the retroperitoneal space. The aneurysm is removed and replaced with a graft in a procedure that takes several hours. Despite the administration of intravenous fluids and many units of blood, his blood pressure falls to 70/40 during part of the surgery.

The following morning the patient is alert and his condition appears stable. His blood pressure is 110/70 as he lies in bed. But he has produced only 50 ml of urine since midnight (confirmed by catheterizing his bladder) and his serum creatinine and BUN have doubled since admission. He has acute renal failure with oliguria—but why?

His physicians consider the possibility that he may have acute tubular necrosis. There are good reasons to suspect this diagnosis. Acute tubular necrosis often occurs following major vascular surgery or severe hypotension, and the patient had both. It is also conceivable that he had a reaction to one of his numerous blood transfusions—another cause of acute tubular necrosis —though there was no clinical evidence of this.

On the other hand, can they be sure that his kidneys are not simply reflecting the effects of poor perfusion? After all, a blood pressure of 110/70 may be less than adequate for a man who has been hypertensive for years. (Even if his pressure were somewhat higher, there could still be doubt about the adequacy of renal perfusion.) Can they be sure that his blood loss has been fully replaced? They can't forget either that this patient does not have a normal heart—another reason renal circulation could be compromised. But the cardiac difficulty also demands caution in administering more blood or intravenous fluids, since too much additional fluid could precipitate acute congestive heart failure.

The physicians squirm a bit; this is a tough problem. Is it really important to know right now whether the patient has tubular necrosis or only hypoperfusion of the kidneys? Emphatically yes! Tubular necrosis means a siege of renal failure that could last for two weeks or more regardless of any treatment, but hypoperfusion usually can and should be treated immediately; it may require nothing more complicated than intravenous fluids to expand plasma volume. Why the hurry? Because prolonged underperfusion of the kidneys may cause this patient to develop acute tubular necrosis if he doesn't have it already.

How can the physicians decide between these two diagnoses? There is no infallible way to make this distinction, but they can get some useful clues. First, they should examine the patient's urine. If his kidneys are simply underperfused but otherwise normal, his urinalysis should be essentially normal except perhaps for some hyaline casts. Even some red blood cells in the urine may not have much significance if the patient has been catheterized or if there is a catheter in his bladder now. But if he has acute tubular necrosis, his urine specimen is likely to show numerous abnormalities, particularly brown pigmented, coarsely granular casts, tubular epithelial cells, free and in casts, and cellular debris.

The physicians may also obtain useful evidence of underperfusion by sending the urine for determination of its sodium concentration and osmolality and its concentration of creatinine relative to that of plasma—the urine-to-plasma (U/P) creatinine ratio. Laboratory experiments with animals have demonstrated that a severely underperfused kidney usually reabsorbs almost all the sodium in its glomerular filtrate, leaving a very low sodium concentration in the urine. It also reabsorbs a large percentage of its filtered water, producing a high concentration of creatinine in the urine compared with the serum. And because of the scant and sluggish flow of tubular fluid through the collecting ducts, which may allow time for some osmotic resorption of water to occur there even in the absence of vasopressin, the hypoperfused kidney sometimes produces a urine significantly hypertonic to plasma.

The kidney with acute tubular necrosis typically does none of these things; its urine usually has a significant concentration of sodium, a low creatinine concentration relative to that of plasma, and osmolality close to that of plasma. Perhaps this is because its tubular cells are too badly damaged to carry out the efficient resorption of sodium and water. Some have suggested that only a few nephrons are still functioning in acute tubular necrosis and that, because of the excretory demands placed on them, these nephrons are behaving as do those in a kidney undergoing osmotic diuresis.

These chemical differences between the typical urine from an underperfused kidney and that from a kidney with acute tubular necrosis are shown in Figure 11-2. Unfortunately, nontypical findings are rather common, and the

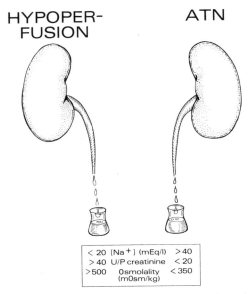

< 20	[Na⁺] (mEq/l)	> 40

< 20	$[Na^+]$ (mEq/l)	> 40
> 40	U/P creatinine	< 20
> 500	Osmolality (mOsm/kg)	< 350

Figure 11-2. Chemical characteristics commonly (but not invariably) found in urine from severely hypoperfused kidneys and from those with oliguric acute tubular necrosis (ATN). The elevation of urine osmolality to hypertonic levels in states of hypoperfusion is a less consistent finding than the other measurements shown. (Data are taken from T. R. Miller, R. J. Anderson, S. L. Linas, et al., *Ann. Int. Med.* 89: 47–50, 1978.)

message may be confusing; what can the physicians conclude if the urine sodium concentration suggests underperfusion of the kidney, but the U/P creatinine ratio is low and the urine is isotonic? Some nephrologists have found it helpful to incorporate some of this same information into a formula that yields a single number instead of two values that may appear to contradict each other. Thus a *renal failure index* can be obtained, calculated as

$$\frac{U_{Na}}{U/P_{creatinine}}$$

This value is 1.0 or less in most cases of hypoperfusion and greater than 1.0 in most cases of acute tubular necrosis. Calculation of the fractional excretion of filtered sodium,

$$\frac{U/P_{Na}}{U/P_{creatinine}} \times 100$$

yields a similar figure, which is interpreted the same way: a value of 1.0 or less suggests underperfusion, whereas a value greater than 1.0 makes acute tubular necrosis likely.

All these guidelines are useful only if oliguria is present and if obstruction of the urinary tract has been ruled out. Renal disease that existed before the onset of acute renal failure may also muddy the picture by causing abnormalities in the urinary sediment and by influencing the osmolality of the urine and its sodium and creatinine concentrations.

If the physicians in charge of our hypothetical patient are still in doubt about the cause of his acute renal failure even after his urine has been scrutinized microscopically and chemically, they may resort to a cautious trial of intravenous fluids or of a potent diuretic such as furosemide. If administration of 500 to 1000 ml (or occasionally more) of isotonic saline solution restores his urinary output, they may reasonably conclude that his oliguric renal failure was on the basis of extracellular-fluid volume depletion. If he has tubular necrosis, he will not respond to the saline, but he will also now have that much extra fluid that he probably didn't need and can't excrete and that may overload his circulatory system. Thus the fluid challenge has its risks.

The furosemide trial is probably a safer approach, provided that the physicians do not lose sight of what is really happening. If 80 mg of furosemide given intravenously causes a marked increase of urine flow, it is likely that the kidneys are underperfused and reabsorbing virtually all of their glomerular filtrate; giving the furosemide has unmasked this situation by blocking the resorption. The physicians must now realize that their patient probably has depletion of the extracellular-fluid volume—which they have just made a little bit worse with their test—and that steps should be taken at once to replenish this fluid space before hypoperfusion evolves into acute tubular necrosis. If the kidneys already have acute tubular necrosis, or if they are so badly underperfused that they are not producing glomerular filtrate, there should be no significant response to furosemide. (Occasionally some response does occur even though the patient has tubular necrosis, causing some authorities to doubt the usefulness of this test.)

A more sophisticated but more invasive way to evaluate the adequacy of the circulating fluid volume is to pass tubes into the vascular system that can be used to measure the pressure in the right atrium (central venous pressure) or, better yet, the "wedge pressure" in the pulmonary circulation, which reflects left atrial pressure. This maneuver should not be considered a routine procedure for the evaluation of acute renal failure—it's rarely necessary, in fact— but in some unusually difficult or confusing situations it has been helpful.

TREATMENT

If acute renal failure is shown to be the result of a postrenal problem, the appropriate treatment is usually quite clear: The obstructed urinary tract must be opened if reasonable and practical means are available, or an alternative route for urinary drainage must be provided. Restoration of urinary drainage typically solves the problem of acute renal failure quite promptly. If prerenal factors are found to be responsible, attention is directed toward restoring adequate circulation to the kidneys. This usually means giving fluids to expand circulating and extracellular-fluid volumes, though occasionally a failing heart must be treated or a vascular obstruction corrected. As in the case of postrenal failure, successful treatment of the cause, if accomplished soon enough, restores renal function quickly.

Acute tubular necrosis is different. This diagnosis implies that an injury to the kidneys has taken place from which they will not recover immediately. They should recover eventually, but in their own good time after some type of healing process has taken place, and there is nothing definitive we can do to speed up the process. So there is really no treatment for the kidneys in acute tubular necrosis.

There is treatment for the patient, however, and it's a real challenge. The object is to keep this person alive despite the absence of renal function for a week or two, longer if necessary, until his own kidneys can take care of him again. The availability of dialysis has taken away some of the stress and suspense that used to accompany this predicament, but it is still a serious situation that demands careful management and has a rather high mortality rate. Most physicians today treat the patient who has acute tubular necrosis with some mixture of what we'll call the predialysis regimen and a newer approach that depends on dialysis. Let's look first at the older method.

In the Bad Old Days

The consequences of abrupt and virtually complete kidney failure are fairly predictable. Unlike the patient with chronic renal failure, who has a significant amount of renal function remaining, a person with acute renal failure is not in a steady state where the output of various substances equals intake. On the contrary, many substances that enter the body keep accumulating there in acute renal failure. Sodium and water are retained, leading to edema, hypertension, and sometimes congestive heart failure. A metabolic acidosis develops because the kidneys can no longer excrete hydrogen ions. Levels of urea and other end-products go higher and higher. As the internal chemical environment deteriorates, the patient becomes more susceptible to infection. But the most threatening change of all is usually the rising level of serum potassium, which can lead to sudden death from cardiac conduction disturbances.

Before dialysis was available to save the patient from this relentless progression of events, there was only one good way to forestall disaster: The patient was not allowed to take in what he could not excrete. Patients with acute tubular necrosis were therefore not allowed to take any sodium, and water was restricted to less than enough to cover insensible losses (see below). Since dietary protein is metabolized to urea, patients were allowed no protein in the diet. Potassium, of course, was poison—none of that could be allowed either. What *could* the patient eat safely? Only pure carbohydrates and fats, since these are metabolized to water and carbon dioxide; the water could be included in the daily allowance, and the lungs would excrete the carbon dioxide. The practical result of these restrictions was a diet of pure carbohydrate and fat: butterballs (butter and sugar) and popsicles (frozen cream and sugar). The patients didn't like this regimen—who would?—but their lives depended on it.

Unfortunately, even these rigid restrictions do not solve all the problems caused by the loss of kidney function, though they help to postpone disaster. The regular turnover of many body protein tissues continues in renal failure and may even accelerate if there has been severe injury; the continuing breakdown of internal proteins leads to formation of urea, release of potassium, and liberation of water. A continuing need for glucose stimulates some of this catabolism (gluconeogenesis), and the rate of tissue breakdown can be slowed by providing at least 100 to 200 g of dietary carbohydrate each day. Since most patients are still in negative caloric balance, a weight loss of 0.3 to 0.5 kg per day should be expected. Failure to lose weight under these circumstances usually reflects a situation in which the expected tissue loss is indeed occurring but in which the patient is retaining extra fluid in its place and becoming overhydrated, while overall weight remains the same. So fluid intake needs to be adjusted downward so that some weight loss will occur. Under these circumstances thirst may be quite strong, though physiologically inappropriate, and patients with acute tubular necrosis have been known to sneak water from flower vases in their hospital rooms!

In addition to the dietary and fluid restrictions just described, the predialysis regimen sometimes included protective isolation; it had been found that serious infections were common in these uremic patients and often contributed to mortality. When the cation-exchange resin, sodium (or calcium) polystyrene sulfonate (known commercially in the United States as

Kayexelate), became available, it provided a means of removing potassium via the gastrointestinal tract and thus extending the length of time these patients could live without kidney function.

Dialysis to the Rescue

The predialysis regimen was a logical one that undoubtedly saved many lives. But basically it was only a stalling tactic; it could delay but not really prevent the consequences of renal failure. Despite anything that could be done, the patient's own metabolic processes would produce enough toxic changes in the internal environment to kill him within a limited time, if kidney function had not recovered first.

The availability of dialysis took away the deadline for recovery of renal function. Though dialysis does not restore a normal chemical state, it produces enough improvement so that a person can be supported indefinitely—until his own kidneys recover, however long that might be.

At first dialysis was employed only to rescue those who appeared to be approaching death from uremia, but the tendency gradually developed to use it much earlier in the course of acute tubular necrosis. Physicians recognized that their patients could be given improved nutritional support and kept in better general condition if dialysis was used more liberally. Though controlled studies were not done, retrospective analysis suggested that patients who were treated with dialysis fairly early in the course of acute tubular necrosis had better survival rates than those who received dialysis only when it became urgently necessary.

The modern approach to acute tubular necrosis includes the use of dialysis relatively early—at least well before florid uremia develops. The availability of dialysis expands treatment possibilities, since drugs and fluids can be administered with the knowledge that (within reasonable limits) they can also be removed from the body. The patient may be given some protein to replace catabolic losses; even intravenous hyperalimentation can be employed if required by his other problems.

Has the rigorous old predialysis regimen been scrapped completely? Not really. Let's remember that dialysis is no picnic, especially in a patient who has other critical problems such as those often associated with acute tubular necrosis. Dialysis in this setting requires invasion of major blood vessels or the peritoneal cavity, and patients with marginal circulatory compensation may not tolerate a hemodialysis treatment. So there are legitimate reasons for physicians to delay dialysis or avoid it completely if they can.

These considerations often result in a compromise that attempts to gain most of the advantages of both the old and new approaches. As soon as acute tubular necrosis is diagnosed, the patient is likely to be placed on the rigid limitations of the predialysis regimen, modified perhaps to allow a small intake of protein. Without these restrictions he might be forced into dialysis within the first few days, which would not otherwise be necessary. And who knows but what this patient may be one of the lucky ones whose tubular necrosis will start to resolve within a few days? If that happens, smart management from the beginning may make it possible to avoid dialysis altogether without jeopardizing the patient. On the other hand, drugs or other treatment that is vitally important for other medical problems need not be withheld because of renal failure, since we can dialyze the patient if and when necessary.

After four or five days the patient is likely to be getting rather azotemic, though still in good condition, and we're getting concerned about his longer-term nutritional needs. Unless there are indications such as increasing urine volume that renal recovery is underway, we may elect to initiate dialysis on a regular schedule at this time, followed by a liberalization of his protein and fluid intake. We still can't throw caution to the winds, since dialysis does not allow complete dietary license, but we can improve a great deal on the old predialysis menu. If the patient's clinical or chemical condition had been deteriorating earlier in his course, we would have started dialysis sooner. Once he is on regular dialysis, we'll plan to continue it until his kidneys recover or until he succumbs to other problems. As in predialysis days, the treatment of acute tubular necrosis is still a waiting game—but now we can wait much longer.

Are There Any Short-Cuts?

Patients and physicians alike would be spared a great deal of trauma and trouble if a way could be found to speed up the recovery of kidneys from acute tubular necrosis. Investigators have been looking for such a treatment, and it has been reported at different times that massive doses of furosemide or intravenous infusions of amino acids reduce the time needed for recovery of renal function. Unfortunately, work from other laboratories and clinical studies have not supported these findings. A recent report from the rat laboratory suggests that infusion of ATP plus magnesium may be helpful, but further work will be needed before this idea can be accepted or rejected. At present we must still focus on treating the patient and let the kidneys recover by themselves when they will.

Can Acute Tubular Necrosis Be Prevented?

As mentioned earlier, the susceptibility of laboratory animals to acute tubular necrosis appears to be reduced if the kidneys are depleted of renin, and this can be achieved by loading the animals with sodium or potassium for two or three weeks. This does not appear to be a practical clinical approach, however. Acute tubular necrosis in people often appears in the wake of disasters, and disasters are usually not predictable. Even within a group of people who are known to be at increased risk of acute tubular necrosis, such as those about to undergo major vascular surgery, most individuals will not develop renal failure, and we can't identify the ones who will. Giving large amounts of sodium or potassium for weeks to the whole group might cause more harm than would the occasional case of acute tubular necrosis that might be prevented.

It does appear, however, that administration of mannitol, an osmotic diuretic, during vascular surgery may reduce the incidence of acute tubular necrosis, and this is now routine practice in some hospitals. The mechanism of protection is not entirely clear. If renal failure is caused in part by tubular obstruction, maintenance of flow through the tubules by means of a diuretic could conceivably keep debris from accumulating and blocking them; or maybe something more subtle is happening.

Experimental evidence suggests that two or more kidney-damaging factors acting together may produce acute tubular necrosis in some situations where one factor alone would not have been sufficient. For instance, impaired renal blood flow and a nephrotoxic agent, each present in a degree or dose that would not by itself cause renal failure, may produce acute tubular necrosis when both are present together. While some of the situations in which tubular necrosis occurs (Table 11-1) are unavoidable, others are potentially preventable. The liability of any patient to acute tubular necrosis may be reduced if we can identify and eliminate correctable risk factors, especially when more than one such factor is present. For instance, a patient who is about to have vascular surgery should not be allowed to become fluid-volume depleted, and nephrotoxic drugs should be avoided if possible.

"Am I Going To Make It, Doc?"

Despite dialysis and other modern methods of support, the overall mortality in acute tubular necrosis is still high. This is not due so much to the renal failure as to the situations in which it usually occurs. A list of the patients who have been treated for acute tubular necrosis in any large center will usually include many of the most disastrous medical, surgical, and traumatic cases in the hospital. While the appearance of acute tubular necrosis in such patients is a serious development that complicates management and may contribute to death, these patients usually do not die—and should not—simply because of renal failure. In fact, when acute tubular necrosis appears in a person who is otherwise in good condition, as happens now and then, the prognosis with competent management is very good.

In short, the prognosis for the patient with acute tubular necrosis is determined largely by what other problems are present.

BIBLIOGRAPHY

E. G. L. Bywaters and D. Beall. Crush injuries with impairment of renal function. *Br. Med. J.* 1: 427–432, 1941.
   The description of air-raid victims that made acute tubular necrosis well known.

J. T. Harrington and J. J. Cohen. Acute oliguria. *N. Engl. J. Med.* 292: 89–91, 1975.

Diagnostic possibilities and approaches in the patient with oliguria.

D. Kleinknecht, P. Jungers, J. Chanard, et al. Uremic and non-uremic complications in acute renal failure: Evaluation of early and frequent dialysis on prognosis. *Kidney Int.* 1: 190–196, 1972.

The retrospective study indicating that patients do better with dialysis.

T. R. Miller, R. J. Anderson, S. L. Linas, et al. Urinary diagnostic indices in acute renal failure. *Ann. Int. Med.* 89: 47–50, 1978.

How to use those chemical determinations on urine to help decide whether the patient has acute tubular necrosis or something else.

J. H. Stein, M. D. Lifschitz, and L. D. Barnes. Current concepts on the pathophysiology of acute renal failure. *Am. J. Physiol.* 234: F171–F181, 1978.

Reviews the different theories and experimental work on the pathogenesis of acute tubular necrosis.

12
Chronic Renal Failure

The scene is a large hospital in 1960. A middle-aged man has just been admitted. He has had kidney disease for many years, characterized by persistent proteinuria, hypertension, and gradually decreasing renal function as measured by chemical tests. However, he felt healthy and carried on a normal life until one year ago, when general lack of energy and a tendency to tire easily forced him to abandon vigorous physical activity. Otherwise, he was able to carry on most of his usual routine until about six months ago. Since then he has felt unwell most of the time. His fatigue has increased, and he has required increasing amounts of sleep. He becomes short of breath on slight exertion. A metallic taste in his mouth has reduced his appetite, and episodes of vomiting have occurred with increasing frequency. He has been admitted to the hospital on two other occasions in recent months for these symptoms, which were treated primarily by dietary modifications with only slight and temporary improvement. Laboratory tests have shown a severe and progressive loss of renal function.

The patient is readmitted now because he has been vomiting frequently and has become less responsive in the past few days. He is somnolent, but arousable, and has a sallow complexion. His respirations are deep and faster than normal, and his blood pressure is elevated. There is slight edema of the legs. The initial plasma chemistry determinations show a very high blood urea nitrogen—the worst he has ever had—and low serum bicarbonate, consistent with metabolic acidosis. His creatinine clearance in the first 24 hours of hospitalization is between 2 and 3 ml/min—about 2% of the expected normal.

Over the next few days the patient's condition deteriorates. He becomes stuporous, rousing only momentarily. On the third hospital day, he begins to have convulsions. The intern watches helplessly; he knows that the patient is suffering from the chemical consequences of advanced kidney failure, which cannot improve because the kidneys now consist largely of scar tissue. In short, the patient is doomed. Following his third convulsion he stops breathing and dies.

The account you have just read summarizes the course and fate 20 years ago of a typical patient with chronic renal failure. Although the rate of progression might vary considerably from one patient to the next, those with this problem faced a more certain prospect of death than most cancer patients. Malignant neoplasms sometimes have remissions, but chronic renal failure only gets worse as more and more kidney tissue is lost without hope of replacement.

Even though advances in medical knowledge and technology have brightened the outlook in the United States and other developed countries, chronic renal failure remains a major problem for patients and for society. The victim is faced with dependence on dialysis, a demanding mode of treatment that only partially replaces normal kidney function. Alternatively, he may accept the risks of renal transplantation. In either case the treatment is neither easy nor certain of success. For the society, the cost of treating people with chronic renal failure is rising at an alarming rate. Approximately 50,000 people in the United States are now on chronic dialysis, and about 4000 kidney transplants are performed each year. The combined cost of these programs, currently over a billion dollars a year, continues to increase.

Dialysis and transplantation will be discussed in Chapters 13 and 14. The point here is that chronic renal failure, which makes such measures necessary and which still kills thousands of people each year, is a big problem, more formidable by far than all other kidney problems combined.

BASIC IDEAS ABOUT CHRONIC RENAL FAILURE

Chronic renal failure is not a specific disease. The term refers to any situation in which there is a permanent reduction of renal function sufficient to cause significant chemical abnormalities in the internal environment. Chronic renal failure may result from many processes, such as most of the specific renal diseases discussed in Chapters 9 and 10. The degree of renal insufficiency and the resulting chemical abnormalities may range from trivial to life-threatening. Unfortunately, chronic renal failure is almost always progressive, since most diseases that are nasty enough to destroy kidney tissue will keep right on doing so until none is left.

Though chemical tests can detect small losses of renal function, the internal environment is usually not sufficiently disturbed to make the patient sick until kidney function is reduced far below normal. As a general rule, a person with 25% or more of normal kidney function is likely to feel quite well. As renal function falls below that level, he may begin to feel "below par" but can generally continue to get along without great difficulties until renal function is reduced to about 10% of normal. At that level he will probably begin to experience significant symptoms of *uremia,* a toxic state caused by retention of waste products. With conservative management, especially dietary modifications, the patient can usually be coaxed along in an acceptable if not vigorous state of health until only 5% of normal function remains. Below that level, life becomes rather miserable, and the patient will deteriorate and die if dialysis or transplantation is not undertaken.

Although various kidney diseases may present differing features in their early stages, with few exceptions they show a striking sameness in their late stages. The clinical picture is dominated by the chemical consequences of inadequate kidney function and the resulting symptoms. Even the morphologic features of individual diseases tend to become obliterated as the kidneys are gradually reduced to a mass of fibrotic tissue. Confronted with the kidney of a patient who has advanced chronic renal failure, the pathologist is likely to take refuge in a diagnosis of "end-stage kidney"—a frank admission that the features of the patient's original renal disease can no longer be identified. Clinicians are equally undiscriminating at this stage; those who care for patients with advanced renal failure often find it difficult to remember what each patient's original renal disease was—because it is no longer important for most decisions. After the house has burned down, it may be impossible to know what started the fire, and such information may be of no practical use to the owner anyway.

The Intact Nephron Hypothesis

An end-stage kidney looks very disorganized: Many glomeruli and tubules have vanished; some of the remaining glomeruli may appear damaged, and the surviving tubules appear distorted as they wind through the scar tissue. It's no wonder that for many years the end-stage kidney was regarded as a non-organ—a structure so devastated that its function could not possibly make any sense physiologically. This concept was challenged in the 1960s by Bricker and his collaborators, who supported their argument with some ingenious laboratory studies. Their experimental design is shown diagrammatically in Figure 12-1. Female dogs were first subjected to an operation to divide the urinary bladder. Each half of the bladder was drained by means of a plastic tube brought out through the abdominal wall, making it easy to collect urine separately from each kidney while the animals were awake. Studies performed at this point, which the authors called Stage I, showed that both kidneys had equal function, as we would expect.

The next step was to damage one of the dog's kidneys in order to produce a lesion similar to that of chronic renal failure in man. This was accomplished by ligating most branches of one renal artery and assaulting the remaining, noninfarcted part of the kidney with mechanical trauma, followed by the injection of bacteria. When recovery from the procedure was complete, renal function was studied again. During this part of the experiment, Stage II, the dog still had one good kidney that was maintaining a normal internal environment. Not surprisingly, all of the functions studied in the damaged kidney were sharply reduced compared with the undamaged kidney. Bricker and his colleagues noted, however, that the glomerular filtration rate and the various tubular functions measured in the impaired kidney were all decreased from normal to about the same degree. So tubular function *per unit of glomerular filtration rate* was about the same in both kidneys. These findings led the investigators to propose the *intact nephron hypothesis,* which suggests that nephrons contributing to the function of a chronically diseased kidney are intact

Experimental   Design

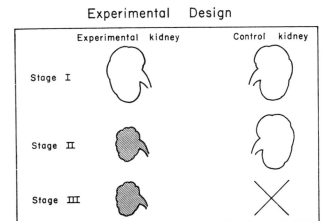

Figure 12-1. Design of experiments to study the functional adaptation of damaged kidneys, using dogs with divided bladders. Stages I, II and III are described in the text. (From N. S. Bricker, E. J. Dorhout Mees, S. Klahr, et al., *Proceedings of the Second International Congress of Nephrology*, Prague, 1963, p. 41. Reproduced by permission of Elsevier/North-Holland Publishing Co.

and working normally, while nephrons that are not intact do not contribute to function at all. In other words, a chronically diseased kidney is characterized by a reduced number of nephrons rather than by malfunctioning nephrons.

Similar results were obtained upon studying some patients who had disease in only one kidney. Figure 12-2 shows the findings in a patient with severe unilateral pyelonephritis.

In the final phase of the dog study (Stage III), the good kidney was removed. Left with only one severely damaged kidney, the dog could no longer maintain a normal internal environment and developed the chemical abnormalities characteristic of chronic renal failure. The behavior of the damaged kidney at this point resembled that of the end-stage kidney in humans. For instance, fractional excretion of sodium became quite high, and a much greater proportion than usual of the glomerular filtrate reached the urine.

If the remaining nephrons of a damaged kidney perform in a normal manner when a healthy kidney is also present (as in Stage II), why do they appear to function differently when the good kidney is no longer present (as in Stage III)? Removal of the opposite kidney does not alter the capabilities of the injured kidney, but it does change the internal environment from a normal one to one with gross chemical abnormalities. It appears reasonable to conclude that damaged kidneys function as they do because of the chemical environment in which they operate, rather than because their surviving nephrons are intrinsically defective.

So the chronically diseased kidney now has a new image. No longer is it seen as battered and helpless. Instead we perceive a small but dedicated population

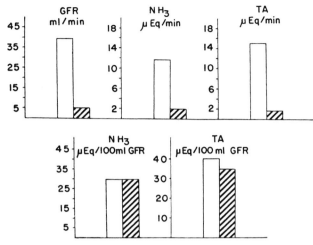

Figure 12-2. Comparison of glomerular filtration rate (GFR), ammonium excretion (NH₃), and titratable-acid excretion (TA) by the kidneys of a patient with unilateral pyelonephritis. Open bars represent the normal kidney, shaded bars the diseased kidney. The three figures in the upper row show absolute measurements that demonstrate a marked reduction of all three functions in the diseased kidney. But if excretion of ammonia or titratable acid by each kidney is divided by the corresponding GFR, as shown in the lower two figures, results are about the same for both kidneys. (Reproduced from N. S. Bricker, E. J. Dorhout Mees, S. Klahr, et al., *Proceedings of the Second International Congress of Nephrology*, Prague, 1963, p. 41. Reproduced by permission of Elsevier/North-Holland Publishing Co.

of intact nephrons battling valiantly to protect the internal environment. They struggle against great odds, a tiny group of survivors trying to carry out the work once done by a large army. They can be only partially successful under the circumstances, and ultimately their effort will fail as they succumb one by one to the dread disease that claimed their companions. But their efforts will have extended the length of time during which a tolerable internal environment could be maintained.

Stated less dramatically, the point here is that the chronically diseased kidney, within its limitations, is doing what needs to be done. For instance, a high fractional excretion of sodium is an appropriate response to a situation in which a few nephrons must eliminate as much sodium as was once handled by many nephrons.

It has been suggested, in fact, that the intact nephron hypothesis should have been called the *adaptive* nephron hypothesis. The idea that all functioning nephrons in the chronically diseased kidney are completely intact actually tends to break down a bit under close scrutiny; they really aren't all totally normal, and it's hard to see how they could be when we look at the structural changes in the end-stage kidney. But the view is still valid that those remaining nephrons approximate normal function and act appropriately.

The Steady State of Chronic Renal Failure

The kidneys play a central role in maintaining the internal environment of normal people in a steady state; that is, they adjust the excretion of water, minerals, and metabolic products in response to intake so that the amount of each of these substances in the body is held constant within fairly narrow limits.

Patients with chronic renal failure also maintain an essentially steady internal state. Their kidneys continue to adjust the output of various substances so that the internal environment, though abnormal, remains fairly stable from one day to the next. Of course, there are gradual changes over an extended period of time as kidney function continues to deteriorate and some substances, such as urea, accumulate gradually. On a given day, however, output is virtually equal to intake. For practical purposes, at least over the short term, the patient can be considered to be in a steady state.

If this is hard to believe, consider what would happen if the patient with chronic renal failure were *not* in a steady state, that is, if the kidneys were unable to excrete much of what is taken into the system. Under such circumstances, there would be a noticeable day-to-day accumulation of various substances, a rather rapid deterioration of the internal environment, and an early demise of the patient. Such events, in fact, typify *acute* renal failure, where the loss of kidney function is virtually complete and the untreated patient may survive for only a week or two. The fact that patients with chronic renal failure can struggle along for months or years reflects their ability to maintain a balance between intake and excretion.

If the patient with chronic renal failure is getting rid of as much sodium, nitrogen, phosphorus, and so on, as he takes in, then why is the internal environment abnormal? Why is there usually excess extracellular fluid, and why are urea and phosphorus levels usually elevated? The fact is that these abnormalities set in motion the mechanisms that make it possible for a small number of nephrons to match the excretory work generally done by a large number of nephrons. For example, expansion of the extracellular fluid volume provides the stimulus that helps a small nephron population to match the sodium excretion of normal kidneys, at least up to a point. Elevation of the blood urea level makes it possible for a few glomeruli to filter a large amount of urea. In each case an equilibrium is reached when internal abnormalities are just bad enough so that the remaining nephrons will increase excretion to equal intake.

Methods of Adaptation to Chronic Renal Failure

We have seen that the chronically diseased kidney can be regarded as having a greatly reduced number of nephrons, that these nephrons maintain a steady state, and that they appear capable of acting in an appropriate adaptive manner.

If a few nephrons handle the excretory chores usually performed by many nephrons, then each surviving nephron in chronic renal failure must be excreting much more of everything than a nephron in normal circumstances. There are only three ways this can be accomplished:

1. Each remaining glomerulus may filter an increased amount of the excretory product. This could be facilitated by an increase in the individual filtration rate of remaining nephrons, which apparently does occur to a limited degree. But the major factor allowing increased filtration per glomerulus of many products is an increase in their plasma concentrations. Such an increase allows more solute to be delivered in each drop of glomerular filtrate. (Chapter 3 explains in more detail how rising plasma concentrations of creatinine balance a loss of nephrons.)
2. The fractional excretion of the product may be increased by decreasing tubular resorption of it from the glomerular filtrate.
3. The tubules may secrete more of the excretory product.

In chronic renal failure, one of these three processes or a combination of them makes possible the increased output per nephron of every substance that depends on the kidneys for excretion. The specific method employed for each substance depends on the way it is normally handled by the kidney.

CHEMICAL CONSEQUENCES OF CHRONIC RENAL FAILURE

The effects of chronic renal failure are only partially understood because our knowledge of what the kidneys do under normal circumstances must be far from complete. Any small molecule in the blood not bound to plasma proteins will be filtered by the glomeruli and, if not reabsorbed by the tubules, excreted in the urine. Numerous such substances have been identified, and surely many more remain undiscovered, especially those present in minute amounts. While some of these excretory products are probably innocuous, others may be toxic, particularly when chronic renal failure causes them to accumulate in the blood. Thus the following account, focusing on some important and well-studied excretory functions of the kidneys, is by no means the whole story of chronic renal failure.

Table 12-1 lists some of the major substances excreted by the kidneys, the principal method(s) by which excretion is maintained in chronic renal failure, important mechanisms or contributing events that help to make this adaptation possible, and some of the clinical consequences of chronic renal failure related to these substances. The comments that follow relate to the table.

Urea

If a patient with chronic renal failure continues to ingest the same amount of nitrogen-containing food as when renal function was normal, plasma urea will rise in rough inverse proportion to the loss of total glomerular filtering

Table 12-1. How a Few Nephrons Do the Work of Many: Methods of Adaptation in Chronic Renal Failure and Some Consequences

Excretory Product	Principal Method(s) of Renal Adaptation	Important Contributing Factors	Clinical Consequences
Urea	↑ Filtered load per nephron	↑ Plasma urea concentration ↑ Flow of tubular fluid per nephron, reducing passive resorption of urea	Elevated plasma urea concentration with resulting morbidity
Creatinine	↑ Filtered load per nephron	↑ Plasma creatinine concentration	Elevated plasma creatinine concentration, which has no evident adverse effects
Sodium	↑ Fractional excretion (↓ % of tubular resorption)	Expansion of extracellular fluid volume, which activates various mechanisms to reduce sodium resorption Possible natriuretic factor Osmotic diuresis in remaining nephrons	Effects of increased ecf volume, such as edema, hypertension, pulmonary congestion
Water	↑ Fractional excretion (↓ % of tubular resorption)	Osmotic diuresis in remaining nephrons Impaired renal concentrating ability Adjustment of vasopressin secretion to needs	Rarely, dehydration More commonly, increased total body water and hyponatremia from limited ability to excrete water
Potassium	↑ Tubular secretion	↑ Flow of fluid and sodium in distal tubules of remaining nephrons Possible ↑K+ content in cells of distal tubule Ability to adjust secretion of aldosterone	Increases of serum K+ in some patients
Phosphorus	↑ Fractional excretion (↓ tubular resorption) ↑ Filtered load per nephron (advanced stages)	↑ Parathyroid hormone (PTH) levels ↑ Plasma phosphorus concentration (advanced stages)	Osteolytic effect of elevated PTH levels Consequences of increased plasma phosphate concentration 1. hypocalcemia 2. promotion of soft-tissue calcification
H+	↑ H+ secretion per nephron 1. ↑ NH₄+ excretion per nephron 2. ↑ titratable-acid excretion per nephron	↑ NH₃ production per nephron, stimulated by acidosis ↑ Phosphate excretion per nephron	Acidosis sufficient to stimulate adequate NH₃ production and H+ secretion Possible demineralization of bones

capacity; filtration and excretion of urea per nephron will increase accordingly. Under normal circumstances, urea accounts for a large proportion (roughly 50%, depending on diet) of the osmotic particles in urine. So when the filtration of urea per nephron is raised manyfold, there is a substantial increase in the total amount of solute each nephron must handle, and the conditions of an osmotic diuresis are created within the remaining nephrons. An increased excretory load per nephron of other solutes contributes to this also, of course.

The presence of an increased osmotic load in the residual nephrons of the chronically diseased kidney has important consequences that are often to the patient's advantage. As the term *osmotic diuresis* implies, resorption of water is impaired, resulting in a high rate of flow in each nephron. One beneficial consequence of this is that an increased percentage of filtered urea is excreted in the urine, since the passive resorption of urea is influenced by the flow of tubular fluid (more flow leads to less resorption). As a result, the rise of plasma urea may be a bit less than would be predicted.

Nevertheless, the rise of plasma urea—blood urea nitrogen (BUN) in American clinical parlance—is one of the most striking features of advanced renal failure. Although urea is not especially toxic, it is not innocuous. Patients with high concentrations of plasma urea usually do not feel well, and may suffer from nausea and vomiting. One hypothesis is that urea in gastrointestinal secretions gets broken down by bacteria to ammonia, which is toxic and irritating to the gut. One of the objectives in the treatment of chronic renal failure is to lower plasma urea levels.

Creatinine

The relatively constant daily internal production of creatinine is excreted almost entirely by glomerular filtration. As glomerular filtration rate falls, the plasma creatinine concentration increases. Thus a steady state can be maintained because the filtered load of creatinine per remaining nephron rises. The increased serum creatinine concentration is useful as an index of renal function but is not harmful to the patient so far as we know.

Sodium

Since plasma sodium concentration does not change markedly or consistently in chronic renal failure, the amount of sodium filtered by each remaining glomerulus can increase only moderately, if at all. Just as in normal subjects, sodium excretion must be regulated by adjusting the resorption of filtered sodium, and this process is sensitive to the volume of the extracellular fluid. The specific intrarenal mechanisms governing sodium resorption were described in Chapter 5. In addition, some researchers have described a natriuretic substance in the blood of subjects with chronic renal failure; its relationship to the postulated natriuretic hormone of nonuremic individuals is not clear at this point. The osmotic diuresis in residual nephrons that is caused primarily by urea also tends to hinder the tubular resorption of sodium and thus to promote its excretion.

Despite these influences, the patient with advanced chronic renal failure often finds it difficult to excrete enough sodium to balance dietary intake and maintain satisfactory internal conditions. When relatively few nephrons remain, the fractional excretion of sodium must be quite high by normal standards, and considerable expansion of the extracellular fluid may be needed to provide the stimulus. But marked expansion of the extracellular fluid can cause problems such as peripheral edema, hypertension, cardiac decompensation, and pulmonary edema, and these are common consequences of renal failure.

Considering the substantial amount of sodium filtered each day by even severely diseased kidneys, it is evident that adequate sodium excretion could be achieved easily if most of the filtered sodium were excreted. But even under the strongest stimuli for sodium excretion it is unusual for more than 20 to 25% of filtered sodium to appear in the urine. The mammalian kidney appears better designed to conserve sodium than to excrete it in large amounts.

Why then are diseased kidneys sometimes described as "sodium wasters"? This label is based on the fact that under conditions of rigid sodium restriction end-stage kidneys may excrete more sodium than normal kidneys. Maybe the osmotic diuresis in residual nephrons is responsible for this phenomenon. Whatever the cause, the obligatory loss of sodium in chronic renal failure is usually small in relation to dietary intake and therefore not a clinical problem. Impaired ability to excrete enough sodium is a far more common problem, one aggravated by the high salt content of the usual American diet.

What has been said here applies to most patients with chronic renal failure, but there are occasional exceptions. Large inappropriate urinary losses of sodium do occur at times in some renal diseases, notably medullary cystic disease. And the problem of sodium retention is not equally severe in all patients with chronic renal failure; those with tubulointerstitial diseases seem less prone to this difficulty than those with glomerular diseases.

Water

Even in severely damaged kidneys the glomeruli supply more than enough filtrate to produce a normal volume of urine if resorption of too much water by the tubules can be prevented. Usually this is no problem because of conditions that favor water excretion and may even require the formation of an increased volume of urine.

As chronic renal failure progresses from early to late stages, there is a gradual loss of the capacity to make hypertonic urine. One reason for this is the fact that the remaining nephrons are undergoing osmotic diuresis. Even normal kidneys stimulated by vasopressin lose the ability to concentrate urine in the presence of large osmotic loads. Presumably the same thing happens in the residual nephrons of chronically diseased kidneys. Even without the osmotic diuresis it is unlikely that damaged kidneys could reabsorb water normally. Production of concentrated urine requires a hypertonic medullary interstitium that is maintained by the efforts of many nephrons and depends on exacting anatomical relationships between various tubular structures and their blood vessels. The medullary architecture in an end-stage kidney reminds one of a bombed-out city—only a few structures remain. It is most unlikely that these few survivors could maintain normal medullary osmolality.

Since normal human urine is moderately hypertonic much of the time, loss of concentrating ability means that most patients will require a greater urine volume than if they were healthy in order to excrete their usual osmotic load. The resulting need to urinate more frequently, especially at night, may be noticeable by the patient and is one of the symptoms of chronic renal failure. However, the daily urine output is not likely to exceed 3 liters unless the patient is excreting an unusual amount of solute (see Chapter 6 and Table 6-1).

As renal disease progresses, the capacity to dilute the urine also becomes impaired, though it tends to be preserved somewhat longer than concentrating ability. Osmotic diuresis in the remaining nephrons may be the cause of this abnormality also.

Late-stage renal disease, thus, is characterized by production of urine with an osmolality that is fixed close to that of plasma. Actually most patients can still vary their urine concentration within a narrow range, presumably in response to vasopressin. So far as we know, the mechanisms for vasopressin release continue to function normally in chronic renal failure, but the ability of this hormone to control water excretion is reduced by the factors at the renal level already mentioned.

Depletion of body water due to an obligatory increase of urine volume is seldom a problem in chronic renal failure because the thirst mechanism is intact and urinary water losses are not extreme. On the other hand, difficulties related to overexpansion of body water are fairly common. Some patients are accustomed to drinking large quantities of liquid. Under normal circumstances this habit results in copious amounts of urine but has no ill effects. When excretion of water is restricted by the limited diluting ability of chronically diseased kidneys, however, a continued high intake of fluid can result in water retention and hyponatremia.

Potassium

Potassium excretion is regulated by tubular secretion, and the capabilities of this mechanism are demonstrated impressively in chronic renal failure. Because of secretory efficiency, homeostasis for potassium and satisfactory serum K^+ levels can usually be maintained to late stages of chronic renal failure. Even patients with 5% of their glomerular filtration remaining can often maintain acceptable serum potassium levels on a normal K^+ intake. This means, of course, that each remaining nephron must be excreting many times its usual output of potassium.

This remarkable performance is possible because many of the influences that favor K^+ secretion (see Chapter 8 and Table 8-1) are usually present in chronic renal failure. Since each surviving nephron is handling many times its regular load of fluid and solute, there is a high flow rate in the distal nephron, and ample sodium is likely to be available for resorption there. If these factors alone are not sufficient to stimulate adequate potassium secretion, plasma and intracellular K^+ may increase somewhat. These changes then stimulate aldosterone secretion and promote transfer of K^+ from cells of the distal tubule into the lumen. We must remember, of course, that aldosterone serves at least two masters, so its secretion may be inhibited in response to expansion of the extracellular fluid volume.

The most important of these influences may be the flow in the distal nephron; this is suggested by the common clinical observation that patients whose daily urine output exceeds 1 liter rarely develop serious hyperkalemia. A significant rise of plasma K^+ above normal levels, though helpful in stimulating potassium secretion, represents a dangerous situation and suggests that other, safer mechanisms of achieving potassium homeostasis have proven inadequate.

Phosphorus

Although phosphorus is a nutrient and an essential constituent of the body, it is also an important renal excretory product. This is because the amount ingested and absorbed (as phosphate ions) each day far exceeds physiological needs.

The day-to-day regulation of phosphate excretion appears to depend on its interaction with calcium, as described in Chapter 2. You will recall that a rise of plasma phosphate tends to produce a fall in plasma ionized calcium, which in turn stimulates the secretion of parathyroid hormone (PTH). PTH then acts on the kidneys to promote the excretion of phosphate. PTH also mobilizes calcium and phosphate from the bone; under normal circumstances, this raises only the serum calcium, since renal excretion of phosphate is being stimulated simultaneously. These relationships and some others to be discussed later are shown in Figure 12-3.

The kidneys process phosphate by glomerular filtration, followed by tubular reabsorption. Under normal circumstances, only about 15% of filtered phosphate reaches the urine, 85% being reabsorbed by an active transport process which takes place largely, if not exclusively, in the proximal tubule. PTH inhibits this resorption.

With this background we can consider the regulation of phosphate excretion in chronic renal failure. As with other excretory solutes, each remaining nephron must excrete much more phosphate than it would under normal conditions if a steady state is to be maintained. This is achieved first by a

Parathyroid Glands

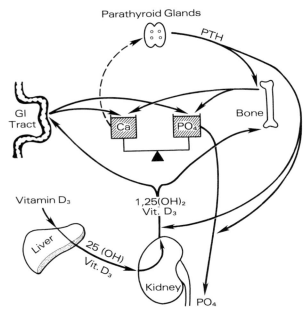

Figure 12-3. Some of the major interactions of plasma calcium (Ca), phosphate (PO₄), parathyroid hormone (PTH), and vitamin D and its metabolites. The dashed arrow represents inhibition of PTH release by high levels of plasma calcium.

reduction in tubular resorption of phosphate, apparently in response to increasing levels of PTH. Figure 12-4 shows in diagrammatic form what is probably happening as renal disease progresses. Each time some nephrons are lost (represented by a reduction of GFR), there is a tendency for plasma phosphate to rise and plasma calcium to fall. The depression of calcium stimulates release of PTH, which decreases renal phosphate resorption and allows plasma phosphate to return to its previous level. A new steady state has been achieved, one that requires higher plasma concentrations of PTH to maintain a higher fractional excretion of filtered phosphate. With each additional loss of nephrons the same sequence is repeated, and the plasma PTH level rises higher.

As renal failure worsens, however, this adaptation eventually breaks down. The time comes when phosphate excretion per remaining nephron cannot be increased any further simply by inhibiting tubular resorption, and additional increases of the plasma PTH titer have little effect. At this point, which is usually reached when about 75% of glomerular filtration has been lost, the plasma phosphorus concentration begins to rise. This increases the filtered load of phosphate per nephron, which, together with continuing inhibition of tubular resorption, makes it possible to maintain a steady state for phosphate.

Unfortunately, the steady state for phosphate is achieved at a price. The plasma concentration of phosphate may reach very high levels, and this may

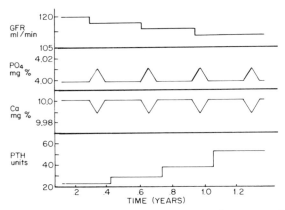

Figure 12-4. Hypothetical representation of the events that cause the plasma concentration of parathyroid hormone (PTH) to increase progressively as renal function decreases. The sequence of events is described in the text. (From N. S. Bricker, E. Slatopolsky, E. Reiss, et al., *Arch. Intern. Med.* 123: 545, 1969. Copyright © 1969, American Medical Association.)

promote the deposition of calcium-phosphate salts in soft tissues. It also tends to depress ionized calcium levels and thus stimulates a huge outpouring of PTH on a chronic basis. The additional secretion of PTH is futile with respect to phosphate excretion, but it can have serious long-term effects on the skeleton, which will be discussed later in this chapter.

Hydrogen Ion (H⁺)

Normal kidneys excrete hydrogen ion by means of tubular secretion; the H^+ appears in the urine as titratable acid (TA) and ammonium (NH_4^+). Patients with chronic renal failure typically excrete nearly as much titratable acid and about half as much NH_4^+ as normal persons on a similar diet. Considering the vastly reduced number of functioning nephrons in chronically diseased kidneys, it is apparent that the output of both TA and NH_4^+ *per nephron* must be increased many times, the increase being somewhat greater for TA than for NH_4^+. How are these increases achieved?

The increase of titratable-acid excretion per nephron is made possible mainly by the increased excretion of phosphate per nephron, which was discussed in the preceding section. To use this additional buffer for H^+ excretion, the residual nephrons must each secrete many times as much hydrogen ion as the nephrons of a normal kidney. They meet the challenge remarkably well, producing urine whose pH is similar to that of normal persons (usually about 6.0). Since the total amount of buffer excreted and the urinary pH are both about normal, the total excretion of titratable acid in chronic renal failure approximates that in health. There is a difference, however; unlike a normal person, the patient with chronic renal failure usually has a significant metabolic acidosis. Given the same degree of acidosis and the same kinds and quantities of solute to be excreted by each nephron, a person with normal kidneys would be likely to produce urine of considerably lower pH (and therefore greater TA). The failure of the chronically diseased kidney to respond in the same way is probably caused by factors in the uremic environment that decrease the resorption of HCO_3^- in the proximal tubule. Biocarbonate that is then passed on to the distal nephron limits acidification of the urine.

A manyfold increase in the excretion of NH_4^+ per nephron is a more complicated achievement, since the sparse population of remaining nephrons must also produce the necessary substrate, ammonia (NH_3). We noted in Chapter 7 that normal nephrons can respond to chronic metabolic acidosis with a great increase in their production of NH_3. Apparently the same phenomenon occurs in residual nephrons when they are exposed to the metabolic acidosis of chronic renal failure; this makes more NH_3 available to be trapped as NH_4^+ in the urine. Though the ability of tubular cells to accelerate NH_3 production is impressive, it is not unlimited, and a severe decrease of functioning renal tissue makes a reduction of total NH_4^+ excretion inevitable. Some recent work indicates that in renal failure there may be an added number of tubular cells in each surviving nephron, but whatever increase occurs is not enough to make up for the nephrons that have been destroyed.

If the excretion of titratable acid is about normal and that of ammonium is definitely reduced, it appears that the kidneys are not maintaining a steady state for hydrogen ion (assuming a normal rate of H^+ production in the body). We might therefore expect the acidosis of chronic renal failure to get progressively worse, but in fact it usually remains stable over long periods of time. Thus there does seem to be a steady state. It is probably achieved by buffering, in the bones, of the H^+ that is not being excreted.

Let's once more consider an old question for a moment: If a patient has achieved a steady state where his urinary output of H^+ plus bone buffering are equal to the dietary load of H^+, why is he acidotic? He is acidotic because he must be in order to reach the steady state. Without the stimulus of acidosis, his tubules would not produce as much NH_3, and H^+ would not be buffered in the bones. The plasma bicarbonate concentration would then fall until worsening acidosis caused enough bone buffering and stimulated the production of enough NH_3 to reestablish a steady state.

Equilibrium for hydrogen ion thus is achieved in chronic renal failure only at the expense of a chronic metabolic acidosis. Over a long period of time, this acidosis may contribute to demineralization of the bones.

OTHER ASPECTS OF CHRONIC RENAL FAILURE

In addition to the specific excretory problems and their consequences that have just been described, the patient with chronic renal failure is likely to experience a number of other difficulties. Some of the more common ones are described below.

Anemia

Most patients with advanced renal failure are anemic, sometimes to a startling degree. Hematocrit values that are one-half of normal or even lower are not unusual. It has been recognized for a long time that production of red blood cells is impaired in uremia, and it seemed reasonable to blame this failure on a shortage of erythropoietin, the hormone that stimulates red-cell production. Erythropoietin is produced in the kidneys, after all, and severely damaged kidneys could hardly be expected to produce adequate quantities of it. Recently, however, using more sensitive assay methods, some investigators have reported that most patients with chronic renal failure have plasma erythropoietin levels that are as high as those of normal people, though lower than those of severely anemic people who do not have renal failure. Some of the fault may lie with the bone marrow, which, even in the presence of erythropoietin, can't produce red cells very efficiently in a uremic chemical environment.

The problem doesn't stop there, however. The red blood cells that are produced have a reduced life expectancy, again probably related to the noxious uremic environment. Patients with renal failure also lose more blood than do normal people because their blood clotting mechanisms may be impaired and because their doctors require numerous blood tests at frequent intervals to see how sick they are.

In short, a patient with chronic renal failure suffers from a combination of decreased production and accelerated destruction or loss of erythrocytes. The severe anemia that results is tolerated surprisingly well by most patients; it is commonplace to see people with hematocrit values of 20% going about their daily activities in a pretty normal manner, though they do not usually engage in strenuous exercise. Their ability to function so well is made possible in part by an increase in red cell 2,3-diphosphoglycerate (2,3-DPG), which lessens the affinity of hemoglobin for oxygen and thus facilitates delivery of oxygen to the tissues. An increase in cardiac output helps also.

There are limits, however, to this remarkable ability to get along with very few red blood cells. If anemia becomes sufficiently severe, patients report disabling fatigue, lethargy, a general sense of ill feeling, and sometimes depression. The degree of anemia necessary to produce these symptoms varies considerably among patients, depending on age and the presence or absence of other medical problems. The authors have observed patients who did not complain until their hematocrits fell to 13 or 14%! Anemia of that severity is unusual in the natural course of chronic renal failure, since people usually die first from other effects of uremia, but it is not rare in patients who are supported by dialysis.

Renal Osteodystrophy

As indicated in the section on phosphate excretion, chronic renal failure leads to elevations of serum phosphate, usually with depression of serum calcium

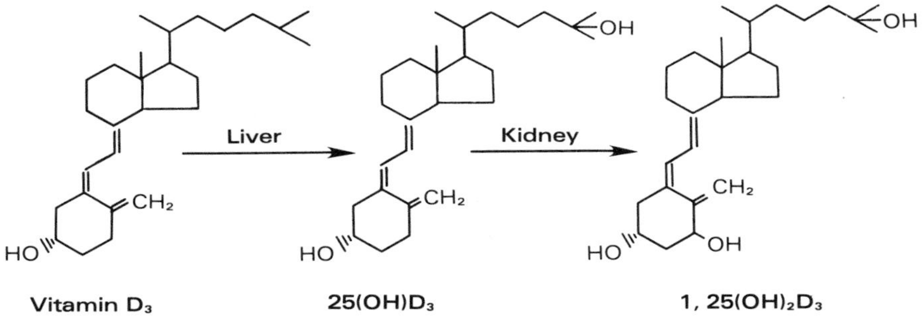

Figure 12-5. Hydroxylation of cholecalciferol (vitamin D_3) to calcitriol [$1,25(OH)_2D_3$] in two stages by liver and kidney.

levels and chronic overproduction of parathyroid hormone. In addition, chronic renal failure has an important direct effect on the activity of vitamin D.

We know now that vitamin D is virtually inactive in the body until it has undergone metabolic conversion. Two hydroxylation steps, the first in the liver and the second in the kidney, change the original compound, cholecalciferol, to 1,25-dihydroxycholecalciferol, or calcitriol (Fig. 12-5). This compound is very potent. Quantities which are measured in micrograms stimulate absorption of calcium from the intestine and affect bone mineralization, so calcitriol is widely regarded now as the active form of vitamin D. Since it is produced in the body, it is properly considered a hormone. Other compounds are also produced by the hydroxylation of cholecalciferol, but their physiological role, if any, is still uncertain.

In chronic renal failure the production of calcitriol is impaired, presumably because there is too little functioning kidney tissue left to carry out the second critical hydroxylation step, and no other organ seems capable of doing this. Though parathyroid hormone promotes the normal renal production of calcitriol, not even the high levels of PTH present in chronic renal failure can stimulate the residual renal tissue to produce enough of it. The consequences to the patient are, in effect, those of vitamin D deficiency. Intestinal absorption of calcium is impaired, contributing to hypocalcemia and impaired calcification of bone. And the lack of calcitriol may have a direct effect on bone mineralization as well. These disordered relationships are shown schematically in Figure 12-6.

So the patient with chronic renal failure is likely to have both excessive levels of parathyroid hormone and a deficiency of calcitriol. The result is often renal osteodystrophy, a bone disorder that has characteristics of both hyperparathyroidism and rickets/osteomalacia, though features of one or the other may predominate in the individual case. Common radiographic features include resorption of bone mineral under the periosteum (often seen best in the fingers), in the clavicles, and in the skull. Areas of increased density

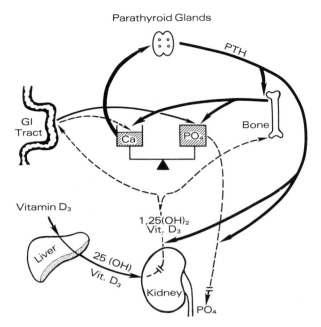

Figure 12-6. The disturbed relationships among plasma calcium, phosphate, parathyroid hormone (PTH), and vitamin D and its metabolites in chronic renal failure. Heavy lines represent the overstimulation of PTH release by low plasma calcium levels and the high concentrations of PTH acting on target organs. Dashed or interrupted lines indicate pathways that are at least partially inoperative or blocked in renal failure. Compare this figure with the normal relationships shown in Figure 12-3.

or sclerosis may appear in the vertebrae, producing the picture of the "rugger-jersey spine." Generalized demineralization may occur, leading to weak bones that are subject to fractures or deformities.

Especially in children the deformities often mimic classical rickets, and the problem has been called *renal rickets.* Since significant renal osteodystrophy usually takes years to develop in adults, it has become more common since chronic dialysis has been used to prolong the lives of those with end-stage renal failure. The patients may be troubled by pain in the affected bones, to say nothing of fractures that may occur with relatively little trauma. Some also have severe muscle weakness.

Neuropathy

Patients with long-standing chronic renal failure often develop dysfunctions of the nervous system, most often involving peripheral nerves. The earliest and most common symptomatic manifestation is a sense of discomfort in the legs if one does not change positions frequently, the so-called "restless-legs syndrome." At this stage there may be no abnormalities on neurological examination, though electronic tests will reveal disturbances in nerve conduction. Later an overt peripheral neuropathy may appear; sensory disturbances such as numbness of the feet are more frequent and usually come earlier than motor weakness. Neuropathy is especially common in those whose renal failure is caused by diabetes mellitus. Such patients are in double jeopardy for this complication, since diabetes mellitus by itself can cause peripheral neuropathy. In those who are not diabetic, serious neurological problems are seen most commonly in patients on chronic dialysis, probably because this group includes those who have lived longest with renal failure.

Despite considerable effort to find a specific chemical abnormality in renal failure that is responsible for neuropathy, the culprit remains unidentified. It seems quite possible that there is no one specific cause. Rather, a number of the abnormalities found in renal failure may be hostile to the delicate cells of the nervous system.

Pericarditis/Pleuritis

In predialysis days, the appearance of a pericardial friction rub was considered a grave prognostic sign in persons with chronic renal failure. It occurred in the advanced stages of uremia and usually heralded the death of the patient within days. Now it is not rare for uremic pericarditis to occur in patients who are maintained on chronic dialysis, and recovery with more vigorous dialysis and/or use of anti-inflammatory agents is the rule. One consequence of pericarditis may be the accumulation of fluid in the pericardial sac; sometimes the effusion is sufficient in amount to cause tamponade, interference with cardiac filling. Months or years after these problems are apparently resolved, postinflammatory changes may result in a chronic constrictive pericarditis, which compromises cardiac function again.

We don't know which of the many chemical abnormalities in chronic renal failure—or what combination of them—causes the pericardium to become inflamed. Some have suggested that viral infections may be partially responsible.

Inflammation of the pleura with pleural friction rubs and/or pleural effusions has also been observed in patients with end-stage renal failure. Presumably the causes—whatever they are—are similar to those of pericarditis.

And the list goes on. Whole books have been devoted to describing and examining the things that go wrong biologically in the presence of chronic renal failure. We have mentioned some of them, selecting those that seem to cause difficulties most commonly for patients and their physicians. There are many other more subtle problems, such as impairment of the clotting mechanism and disturbance of carbohydrate metabolism, which we will not attempt to deal with here. It is useful to remember, however, that chronic renal failure results in a host of abnormalities in the internal environment, and all of the cells in the body are likely to be affected to some degree. As one investigator expressed it, "Nothing works right in a uremic environment."

How the Patient Feels

In describing the objective abnormalities that characterize chronic renal failure, we referred briefly to some of the associated symptoms. These vary a great deal, depending on the age and general strength of the patient and the presence or absence of other serious medical problems. Some people insist that they feel fine and carry on with vigorous activities despite laboratory evidence of far-advanced renal failure. Others feel unwell at stages where the changes in body chemistry are much less severe.

Nausea, a metallic taste in the mouth, and vomiting are among the most frequent symptoms associated with the uremic state. They are often intermittent, allowing the patient to maintain a reasonable intake of food despite unpredictable bouts of emesis. General lethargy and fatigue are common also. A combination of severe anemia, acidosis, and fluid retention is likely to make the patient dyspneic on exertion and sometimes even at rest. Many persons with chronic renal failure are troubled greatly by intractable itching, which may be related to deposition of calcium phosphate salts in the skin or directly to high levels of parathyroid hormone. We have already mentioned the problem of restless legs. Women with advanced chronic renal failure usually have irregularities or complete cessation of menstrual periods due to disturbances of hormonal regulation. Men suffer from impotence, which is probably more related to general lack of well-being than to specific hormonal deficiencies.

In terminal stages, the picture described at the beginning of this chapter develops. Somnolence and mental confusion progress to stupor and coma, sometimes with convulsions.

TREATMENT OF CHRONIC RENAL FAILURE

There is nothing mysterious about the treatment of chronic renal failure. If one understands the normal role of the kidneys and the disturbances that result when their function is impaired, most of the treatment becomes self-evident.

Diet

The excretory job of the kidneys consists largely of protecting us from the consequences of eating and drinking. Even a wholesome diet provides many substances that will upset the internal environment if they or their metabolic products are not excreted by the kidneys. As we have seen, damaged kidneys continue to cope with this challenge, but the conditions necessary to produce the needed level of output may be distinctly detrimental. So it makes good sense to reduce the excretory demands on the damaged kidneys by modifying dietary intake. Because kidney failure does not have exactly the same consequences for everyone, the diet must be tailored to the demonstrated needs and renal capabilities of each patient. The following generalizations, although roughly applicable to most people with chronic renal failure, must be individualized.

In the early stages of chronic renal failure, no dietary limitations are usually necessary. The patient is likely to feel quite well. He may have no hypertension or evident fluid retention, the level of plasma urea may be too low to cause morbidity, and the plasma concentrations of potassium and other electrolytes are likely to be normal. Then why burden this person with unnecessary restrictions?

As renal failure progresses, however, it is usually important to limit dietary sodium and protein. Sodium is restricted if the patient is hypertensive or has edema or other signs of fluid retention. Reducing protein intake helps to keep the blood urea nitrogen (BUN) concentration at acceptable levels. No one knows exactly what acceptable levels are, but many patients seem to feel less well after the BUN rises above 80 mg/dl (though admittedly some people tolerate twice that concentration). Dietary protein also gives rise to fixed acid and is a rich source of phosphorus, so protein reduction helps to alleviate acidosis and decreases the amount of phosphate that needs to be excreted. Extreme protein restriction (to 20 g daily) is rarely practiced in the United States now, since most people would rather be on chronic dialysis treatments than on such a diet, which is extremely limited. In times and places where dialysis was not generally available, however, severe protein restriction has proved a useful means of prolonging life in renal failure. When so little protein is eaten, care must be taken to see that nutritionally adequate amounts of essential amino acids are provided.

As we have seen, most patients can maintain acceptable plasma levels of K^+ until the very late stages of chronic renal failure, so limitation of potassium intake need not be an automatic part of management. When the plasma K^+ concentration begins to rise, a reduction of potassium intake becomes appropriate. Restriction of protein foods will already have curtailed an important dietary source of potassium.

Though many nervous physicians routinely limit the amount of fluid allowed to the patient with chronic renal failure, this is often unnecessary. Of course, chronically diseased kidneys cannot excrete water as well as normal kidneys, but they can often do it well enough to handle whatever a reasonable person would be likely to drink. We can use the same rule here that we apply to other situations: If the serum sodium concentration is normal, the patient is coping well with whatever amount of water he is drinking and does not need another restriction to burden his life. But if there is hyponatremia, this indicates that the patient is accumulating water (assuming, of course, that he is not sodium-depleted) and that his fluid intake should be reduced.

Fluid and Blood Pressure Problems

Limiting sodium intake is the most physiological way to control the accumulation of excess extracellular fluid. Unfortunately, this approach is not always effective, either because the patient's kidneys can excrete very little sodium or the patient is unwilling to forsake salty food, or for both reasons. Diuretics may be of some help in promoting sodium excretion, though they tend to be less effective as the patient progresses toward advanced renal failure. Perhaps this is because the individual's surviving tubules are already being prodded close to the limits of their sodium-excreting capacities by potent internal stimuli. Even furosemide or ethacrynic acid may have little effect in the usual doses, although a response can sometimes be achieved with huge amounts. It is not a very satisfactory situation, since large quantities of drug must be given—at the risk of toxic effects—to achieve a small increase in sodium excretion.

Patients with limited cardiac reserve may be tipped into congestive failure and pulmonary edema by relatively little fluid retention. In addition to removal of the excess fluid, which is difficult to accomplish in chronic renal failure, digitalis glycosides may help to support the heart. Since many of these drugs or their active metabolites are excreted by the kidneys, doses must be reduced in the presence of significant renal failure.

The high blood pressure so common in renal failure will often respond to effective control of fluid accumulation. Hypertension remains a vexing problem in many patients, however, because fluid accumulation cannot always be controlled or because an outpouring of renin from the damaged kidneys results in peripheral vasoconstriction. Those with this problem can usually be treated with the same antihypertensive drugs used in patients who do not have kidney failure.

Calcium, Phosphorus, and Bone Problems

The need to maintain phosphorus excretion with a decreasing number of nephrons leads to the problems we have described: increasing concentrations of parathyroid hormone, with resulting damage to the bones, and eventually elevated levels of serum phosphate, which may depress the serum calcium and predispose to soft-tissue calcification. Restriction of dietary phosphate intake would be a logical way to avoid this problem, and this approach works well in laboratory animals with renal failure. It has been a flop in humans, however, because a diet that is really low in phosphorus is impractical and unacceptable to most people. Significant amounts of phosphorus are found in so many foodstuffs that its exclusion leaves one with very little to eat.

So an alternative approach to the phosphorus problem is commonly used. If we can't keep people from eating it, maybe we can keep them from absorbing it from the intestine. This is done by giving large amounts of aluminum hydroxide or aluminum carbonate, commonly used antacids.

When the aluminum meets phosphate in the gastrointestinal tract, aluminum phosphate is formed. This compound is virtually insoluble and nonabsorbable, so phosphate that would have been absorbed is excreted with the stools instead. This chemical exchange in the gut also leaves behind a hydroxyl or carbonate ion that helps to reduce the metabolic acidosis of renal failure.

The use of aluminum-containing antacids is a fine idea, but it has some real limitations. Many patients dislike the taste or texture of the aluminum compounds, whether in tablet or liquid form, and would rather risk the long-term consequences of phosphate retention than take these medications. Aluminum compounds also cause constipation, which can be severe in some patients. Antacids formulated for nonrenal patients often include a laxative magnesium compound to counter the constipating effect of the aluminum, but magnesium ion can be absorbed and accumulated to toxic levels in patients with severe renal failure, so it isn't used in such patients. In short, the measures available to treat phosphate retention in chronic renal failure leave much to be desired.

Another facet of the calcium-phosphate problem in chronic renal failure is the impaired ability to convert vitamin D to its active form, calcitriol. It has been possible to overcome this problem in some patients by giving vitamin D in massive doses, but this approach has some drawbacks. Conventional vitamin D has a long half-life; therefore, its full effect may not be apparent for some time, and an overdose results in hypercalcemia that may persist for weeks or longer. Synthetic calcitriol, which has recently become available for clinical use, acts rapidly and briefly and so appears to be a safer and more satisfactory drug. It has already proved its usefulness in many patients with renal osteodystrophy, most notably in children. It does not solve the phosphate retention problem, however, and it is dangerous to use calcitriol or other vitamin D compounds in patients whose phosphate levels cannot be held near normal. Raising the plasma calcium in the presence of a high phosphate level probably sets the patient up for soft-tissue calcification.

Anemia

There is no uniformly effective treatment for the anemia of chronic renal failure. Synthetic erythropoietin is not available, and even if it were, we are not sure that it would work in the uremic environment. Various androgenic hormones have been used to stimulate erythrocyte production; they seem to raise the hematocrit modestly in some patients and have no impact at all on others. They also have some side effects such as increased fluid retention and undesirable hair growth, and sometimes they cause cholestatic jaundice. (Androgenic hormones have also been used in male patients as treatment for impotence. Some patients claim to be helped, but many are not. Skeptics claim that the major benefit is psychological from the knowledge that one is taking sex hormones.)

It is easy to forget that patients with renal failure may have other reasons for their anemia such as blood loss, iron deficiency, and vitamin deficiencies. These causes, some of which can be treated effectively, should not be overlooked. Another common mistake is to give blood transfusions for degrees of anemia that are well tolerated by the patient, although alarmingly low by normal standards. There are some patients, however, for whom repeated transfusions are necessary in order to maintain an acceptable quality of life.

Other Challenges

As we have already mentioned, uremic pericarditis and pleuritis may respond well to anti-inflammatory agents such as indomethacin; such drugs may cause worsening of renal function and should be used with caution. Pericarditis and pleuritis are often associated with severe uremic disturbances of the internal environment, however, and their appearance calls for reexamination of the patient's general status. If the patient is already being supported by dialysis, he may not be receiving enough treatment. If he is not yet on dialysis, perhaps he should be.

A moderate degree of chronic metabolic acidosis is usually accepted as unavoidable. What is there to do that is not being done already for other reasons? Restriction of dietary protein has lessened the excretory load of fixed acid, and the aluminum antacids used as phosphate binders neutralize some H^+. A few patients can be treated with sodium bicarbonate, but most people with chronic renal failure already have more sodium than is good for them. Potassium bicarbonate might overwhelm the already strained excretory capabilities for K^+. Fortunately, chronic acidosis, if not severe, is well tolerated.

There is no simple solution for the intractable itching that plagues many patients. Hot or cold baths and topical ointments and creams are used with partial success, as are systemic antipruritic drugs (which usually make the patient sleepy). Repeated exposure of the affected areas to ultraviolet light has met with some success, but this method is time-consuming and expensive and provides only temporary relief.

Since the specific cause of uremic neuropathy is unknown—it may be multifactorial—there is not much to be done about this except for the measures that have already been discussed to keep the internal environment as close to normal as possible. As is true in the case of anemia, causes other than renal failure (e.g., vitamin deficiencies, drug toxicity) must be considered and eliminated when found.

Skillful direction along the lines described here—with the cooperation of the patient, of course—can improve the quality and length of life in the person with progressive renal failure. Brains can be substituted for nephrons, up to a point. But eventually, with the continuing loss of nephrons, the time comes when a tolerable internal environment can no longer be maintained even with the best management. At this point the patient sinks into the pattern of terminal uremia and dies, unless a substitute for kidney function is provided.

Fortunately, substitutes for one's own kidneys are now available. Despite their limitations, dialysis and renal transplantation have become very important in the treatment of chronic renal failure and have saved thousands of people from otherwise certain death. These methods of treatment will be described in the following chapters.

BIBLIOGRAPHY

N. S. Bricker. On the pathogenesis of the uremic state. *N. Engl. J. Med.* 286: 1093–1099, 1972.

N. S. Bricker, P. A. F. Morrin, and S. W. Kime, Jr. The pathologic physiology of chronic Bright's disease. An exposition of the "intact nephron hypothesis." *Am. J. Med.* 28: 77–98, 1960.

J. W. Coburn. Renal osteodystrophy. *Kidney Int.* 17: 677–693, 1980.

H. F. DeLuca. Recent advances in our understanding of the vitamin D endocrine system. *J. Lab. Clin. Med.* 87: 7–26, 1976.

S. Giovannetti and G. Barsotti: Uremic intoxication. *Nephron* 14: 123–133, 1975.

M. A. Holliday, K. McHenry-Richardson, and A. Portale. Nutritional management of chronic renal disease. *Med. Clin. North Am.* 63: 945–962, 1979.

J. P. Naets. Hematologic disorders in renal failure. *Nephron* 14: 181–194, 1975.

N. H. Raskin and R. A. Fishman. Neurologic disorders in renal failure. *N. Engl. J. Med.* 294: 143–148 and 204–210, 1976.

E. Slatopolsky and N. S. Bricker. The role of phosphorus restriction in the prevention of secondary hyperparathyroidism in chronic renal disease. *Kidney Int.* 4: 141–145, 1973.

13
Dialysis

In chemical terms, dialysis is a process in which water and solute molecules diffuse through a semipermeable membrane from an area where their concentration is higher to one where their concentration is lower. The principle was discovered more than a century ago, when chemists observed that water and small molecules can move through certain membranes that hold back larger molecules. Only in recent decades, however, have advances in technology and medicine made it practical to apply this principle to the treatment of kidney failure.

As we have seen, renal failure is characterized by an increased concentration in the patient's plasma of many substances that depend on the kidneys for excretion. Among the most obvious of these are urea, phosphate, and sometimes potassium. In clinical dialysis, we arrange a situation where the patient's blood is on one side of a semipermeable membrane. On the other side is a solution, the *dialysate,* that lacks these substances or (in the case of potassium) contains them in lower concentration than in the plasma. Because of their concentration gradients, more molecules of urea, phosphate, and potassium pass from the patient's plasma into the dialysate than go in the opposite direction (Fig. 13-1). When the concentration of these products in the dialysate increases to equal that in the plasma, diffusion becomes equal in both directions and net removal from the plasma ceases. But before that point is reached, the dialysate can be thrown away and replaced with fresh solution, allowing the cleansing of the blood to continue.

The semipermeable nature of the membrane is very important. This keeps the patient's albumin and larger protein molecules from being lost into the dialysate, to say nothing of red blood cells, white blood cells, and platelets.

Even in the uremic patient there are many substances in the plasma whose concentrations usually are not elevated and whose large-scale removal would be harmful. Among these are sodium, chloride, calcium, and glucose. Loss of these solutes is prevented by adding them to the dialysate in concentrations approximately equal in those in normal plasma. Their diffusion across the membrane then will be about equal in both directions, and no net loss will occur.

Dr. Michael Madden was a coauthor of this chapter.

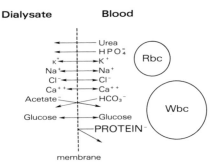

Figure 13-1. Diagram showing some of the exchanges across the semipermeable membrane during a dialysis treatment. $HPO_4^=$ represents phosphate in its usual form at the pH of blood. Red blood cells (Rbc) and white blood cells (Wbc) are far too large to traverse the membrane, as are most protein molecules.

The composition of a typical dialysate solution for hemodialysis is shown in Table 13-1. In many respects it is like normal extracellular fluid—with the omission of solutes like urea and phosphate, which the patient needs to eliminate as much as possible. Potassium is present in reduced concentration because of the need to remove some K^+ from the patient; if this need is urgent, K^+ can be left out of the dialysate completely. You may also have noticed the absence of bicarbonate in the dialysis solution and its replacement by acetate. This is done for purely practical reasons, because it's somewhat difficult to prepare stable solutions with bicarbonate. When an acetate ion diffuses into the patient's plasma, it is metabolized by the liver, resulting in the formation of a bicarbonate ion. Usually this more than balances the bicarbonate ions that diffuse out of the plasma. So plasma bicarbonate usually rises with dialysis—a good thing, since most patients with renal failure have a metabolic acidosis.

The rate at which a solute can be removed by dialysis depends not only on its molecular characteristics and its concentration gradient across the membrane but also on the surface area available. In practical terms, this means that a big membrane area is needed in order to perform an effective dialysis treatment. Despite many ingenious and even bizarre approaches to this problem (such as using the pleural space or the vagina), as yet only two adequate membranes have been found:

Table 13-1. Formulation of a Typical Dialysis Solution

Solute	Concentration (mEq/liter)
Sodium	132
Chloride	104
Potassium	2.0
Calcium	3.5
Magnesium	1.5
Acetate	35
Glucose	11 (200 mg/dl)

1. An artificial membrane, external to the body, so arranged that the patient's blood flows past one side of the membrane and dialysis solution past the other. The membrane can be made as large as necessary. When such a membrane is used, the process is called *extracorporeal* (literally, outside the body) *hemodialysis*—or more simply, just *hemodialysis*. The popular term for this membrane and the necessary supporting equipment is the *artificial kidney*.

2. The peritoneum, a membrane that lines the peritoneal cavity and envelops all the organs in it. The blood supplying the peritoneum is separated from the peritoneal (abdominal) cavity by only two layers of cells in many places. This is conducive to efficient diffusion of solutes from the blood into dialysate, which can be placed in the peritoneal cavity. But the large size of the peritoneal membrane—estimated at 1.5 to 2.0 square meters in an average adult—is the most compelling reason for its choice. Dialysis using this membrane is called *peritoneal dialysis*.

There were major obstacles to the use of each of these systems of dialysis, problems so formidable that at least a partial answer to them had to be found if the method was to be used clinically. Despite the solutions that have been developed, both forms of dialysis still pose problems that can frustrate physicians and their patients alike. We shall describe the major obstacles, solutions, and remaining problems briefly in the following sections.

HEMODIALYSIS

The Obstacles

The three major obstacles to the use of hemodialysis were the need for a suitable membrane, clotting of the blood, and the requirement of adequate access to the patient's vascular system.

Hemodialysis requires a membrane that allows the easy passage of small water-soluble molecules (but not large ones), that can be made thin enough to permit efficient transfer, is chemically inert, is not thrombogenic (i.e., does not stimulate the clotting system), can be sterilized, and can be manufactured to consistent specifications. Regenerated cellulose, a cellophanelike material, has been found to possess these qualities to a satisfactory degree and is now used in almost all available dialyzers. The membrane has a thickness of only about 15 microns and provides a surface area ranging (in dialyzers for adults) from 0.6 to 2.5 square meters. Whereas early dialyzers had to be very large in order to provide the necessary surface area, modern dialyzers are quite compact (Fig. 13-2). The reduction in size is often made possible by a sandwich type of design in which thin layers of blood and dialysate flow past each other (Fig. 13-3). In other dialyzers the blood flows through coils or hollow fibers of membrane material that are surrounded by dialysate.

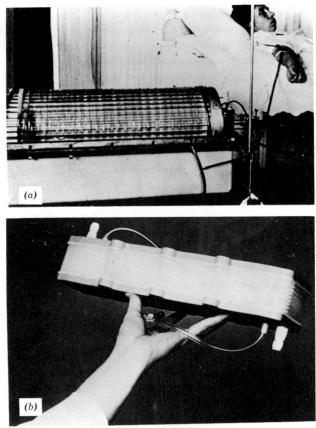

Figure 13-2. (*a*) Early dialyzer developed by Kolff (mid-1940s). (*b*) Modern parallel-plate dialyzer. (Photographs were provided by Mr. Patrick McBride of Travenol Laboratories.)

The introduction to clinical use of the anticoagulant heparin did much to make hemodialysis possible. Clotting mechanisms are activated whenever blood is removed from the body, even when it is in contact with relatively nonthrombogenic membrane material. If coagulation of blood occurs, it will clog the channels in the dialyzer and prevent return of the blood to the patient. Heparin can inhibit such clotting, but its dose must be adjusted

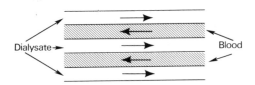

Figure 13-3. Basic design of a parallel-plate dialyzer, seen in side view. Only a few layers, or plates, are shown here; many more are used in a dialyzer.

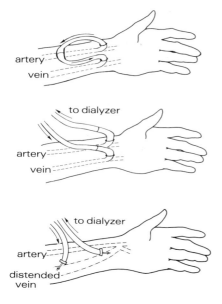

Figure 13-4. Arrangements for repeated access to the circulation. The upper drawing shows an arteriovenous shunt when not in use. Blood flows through the tubing from artery to vein. Note that the two arms of the loop are separate, connected by a coupling. In the middle figure the coupling has been taken apart and the arms connected to the dialyzer by means of tubing. The lower drawing illustrates a subcutaneous arteriovenous fistula into which needles have been inserted to carry blood to and from the dialyzer.

carefully. With too little heparin, blood will clot in the dialyzer. Too much heparin may cause the patient to have a serious hemorrhage.

Hemodialysis requires that 150 to 250 ml of blood be removed from the patient every minute, run through a dialyzer, and then returned to the circulation. Ordinary veins will not deliver blood at this rate, so access to a greater blood flow is needed. The first hemodialysis treatments in humans were carried out by inserting tubing surgically into an artery and an adjacent large vein. After the treatment the vessels were tied off, and another site was used for the next treatment. This limited the use of hemodialysis to patients with acute, reversible renal failure whose kidneys could be expected to recover before their blood vessels were used up.

Development of easy access to the circulation on a repeated basis was the last major development in allowing the use of long-term hemodialysis. In the early 1960s Scribner and Quinton introduced the arteriovenous shunt, a loop of nonthrombogenic plastic tubing that carried blood from an artery (usually in the forearm) out through the skin and then back into a vein. A coupling on the external part of the loop could be disconnected in order to pass the blood through a dialyzer (Fig. 13-4). The continuous flow of blood through the loop at other times helped to discourage clotting in it, and meticulous local care was employed to inhibit infection where the tubing passed through the skin.

The internal arteriovenous fistula introduced by Cimino and his colleagues represented a further advance and is now the most frequently used method of establishing vascular access. With anastomosis of an artery, usually the radial artery in the nondominant wrist, to a neighboring vein, arterial pressures are transmitted to the vein. The vein is gradually transformed into a huge, superficial vessel that provides the blood flow needed for hemodialysis and is easily entered with large needles (Fig. 13-4). Except during dialysis, the blood does not flow through any foreign material, and the vessel is under the skin, so the risks of clotting and infection are greatly reduced.

Substitutes for veins have been used in patients in whom a good fistula cannot be created by a simple anastomosis. Occasionally, a segment of saphenous vein from the leg is tunneled superficially under the skin of the forearm and connected to the radial artery at one end and the deep veins at the other. More frequently, a segment of bovine carotid artery or a synthetic material is used.

The Procedure

Preparation of the dialysis machine takes 20 to 60 minutes; plastic tubing must be fitted to the proper connections under aseptic conditions, and the blood circuit must be primed with a sterile solution of isotonic saline. The patient then sits in a comfortable reclining chair next to the dialysis equipment, and his vascular access is connected with the lines to the dialyzer. If he has an arteriovenous fistula, this is accomplished by introducing two large needles through the skin into the fistula. Heparin is added to the blood to prevent clotting. A roller pump propels the blood through the dialyzer at a rate of about 250 ml/min, while another pump moves prewarmed dialysate through, usually in a countercurrent direction, at about 500 ml/min. A four-hour treatment will use 120 liters of dialysate. The patient's blood pressure and pulse are checked at regular intervals, often by the patient himself, who may also watch the gauges that monitor flows and pressures in the machine.

As we have seen, patients with chronic renal failure often accumulate sodium, but this does not raise the serum sodium concentration because water is also retained. The net result is an excess of extracellular fluid, including plasma volume, which needs to be removed just like other retained products. The removal of plasma water together with its small solutes is known as ultrafiltration. Ultrafiltration is accomplished in hemodialysis by creating a pressure gradient across the dialyzer membrane. Water is then forced across the membrane, carrying the small solutes with it and leaving behind larger solutes and cellular elements. This process is analogous to ultrafiltration by the normal human glomerulus, and it removes a solution of similar composition from the circulation. Pressure across the membrane can be exerted either by increasing the hydrostatic pressure in the blood compartment or by applying suction to the dialysate compartment. It is often possible to remove 1 liter or more of plasma water for each hour of treatment.

Most patients with chronic renal failure require both dialysis of waste products and ultrafiltration of plasma water, but sometimes one form of treatment is needed much more than the other. Methods are available to carry out these two processes together or independently, using the same dialyzer.

A typical patient on long-term maintenance hemodialysis receives three treatments a week, each one lasting four to six hours. Not long ago hemodialysis was considered such a complex and heroic procedure that a doctor and nurse had to be in constant attendance. Now quite a few patients have dialysis machines in their homes and have been trained to carry out their own treatments, usually with some help from a family member. Hemodialysis has become simpler, and most patients are more capable of doing such things than we once thought. Excellent results are usually achieved with home dialysis, which gives the patient a sense of participation and independence and also saves a great deal of money for whoever is paying the bill. It is unfortunate that most patients are still treated in hospitals or in dialysis centers.

Problems Directly Related to Hemodialysis

Although many patients can undergo repeated hemodialysis treatments for months or years without significant difficulties, the procedure carries the inherent risk of some problems that can be very trying.

Threats to Vascular Access

Regardless of the type of vascular access used, infections and clotting are major potential complications feared by all dialysis patients. A well-cared-for fistula or graft can remain functional for many years. On the other hand, there are some patients for whom hemodialysis has become impossible because of failure to achieve or maintain adequate access to the circulation. If these patients are not candidates for peritoneal dialysis or immediate transplantation, their very lives are threatened by the loss of this lifeline.

Bleeding and Blood Loss

The necessary use of heparin to prevent blood from clotting in the dialyzer and blood tubing predisposes the patient to bleeding complications. In some cases this can be extremely serious as, for example, in the patient with underlying ulcer disease or in a diabetic who is prone to retinal hemorrhages. There have been many methods used to minimize the amount of anticoagulation the patient receives, but this is a double-edged sword because it is also undesirable to lose blood by clotting the dialyzer, especially if it happens repeatedly. Even under the best of circumstances a small amount of blood is left in the dialyzer with each treatment. This continuing loss might be insignificant to a normal person, but it is a threat to the dialysis patient who, like other persons with chronic renal failure, often suffers from severe anemia.

Disequilibrium, Hypotension and Cramps

A four-hour dialysis treatment must remove excretory products that have accumulated for two or three days. This results in rather abrupt changes in the internal environment, such as a sharp drop in urea concentration, a change in pH, and loss of plasma volume. It is hardly surprising that some patients become ill during their treatments. Such difficulties often appear related to the fact that plasma water, which is directly affected by the dialysis, does not equilibrate immediately with other compartments in the body.

In its most serious form, dialysis disequilibrium can cause coma, seizures, or death. More common manifestations are nausea, vomiting, headache, hypertension, or transient mental changes. These symptoms may develop while the patient is still on dialysis or within a few hours afterward. They may last for several hours, with subtle effects such as uncharacteristic behavior or headaches lasting for up to 24 hours or more. The exact cause is not entirely clear, but the symptoms seem to stem from cerebral edema and intracranial hypertension. Although severe disequilibrium can be treated, the problem is best avoided by deliberately performing a shorter and less efficient dialysis on patients who are at unusual risk, especially those with very high plasma urea concentrations.

Hypotension during dialysis is a common and occasionally life-threatening problem. Usually it reflects the removal of plasma water—essentially a loss of circulating volume—in excessive amounts or at a rate faster than it can be replaced from edema fluid in the tissues. Other problems such as cardiac disease, autonomic neuropathy, and intolerance to the acetate in the dialysate may limit the ability of the cardiovascular system to maintain blood pressure in the face of plasma-volume losses. When hypotension occurs, patients are placed in a feet-up, head-down position, and, if necessary, given saline solution intravenously.

Some patients experience muscle cramps during dialysis treatments. This is probably another manifestation of acute plasma-volume reduction.

Hepatitis

Outbreaks of hepatitis have occurred in some dialysis centers, spreading from one patient to another and to personnel, who can easily become exposed to the blood of many patients in a day's work. Blood products, which are used frequently, are another potential source of infection. Patients suspected of harboring hepatitis virus are isolated, and many dialysis units will not accept a patient who is believed to be a hepatitis carrier.

Dementia

In some long-term hemodialysis patients, a relentless neurological deterioration has appeared, progressing gradually from gait disturbances and stuttering speech to mental changes, unresponsiveness, and death. The cause is unknown, and the incidence is highly variable from center to center. According to one theory, this syndrome may be related to high levels of aluminum in the brain.

PERITONEAL DIALYSIS

The Obstacles

Peritoneal dialysis could not be employed clinically until means became available to deal with peritonitis, or infection of the peritoneal cavity. It was shown 50 years ago that peritoneal dialysis prolongs the survival of dogs with severe renal failure. Placing a tube through the body wall into the abdominal cavity incurs a substantial risk of infection, however, and many of these animals got peritonitis. In those preantibiotic days, peritonitis was usually fatal, so peritoneal dialysis was simply too risky to use in humans. Peritonitis is still a serious problem, of course, but modern antibiotics make its treatment possible.

At one time peritoneal dialysis was prohibitively cumbersome. Sterile solutions of the proper concentration had to be mixed and introduced into the peritoneal cavity through rubber tubing, which caused problems due to tissue reaction. The availability of inert plastic tubing and premixed solutions in sterile containers did much to make peritoneal dialysis a practical procedure, as did new techniques for placing the tubing into the abdominal cavity.

The Procedure

Before peritoneal dialysis can be carried out, a specially designed catheter must be placed into the abdominal cavity. This procedure can be carried out at the patient's bedside using local anesthesia and scrupulous sterile technique. If only one or two dialysis treatments are anticipated, a temporary catheter is inserted straight through the abdominal wall. If repeated dialysis treatments are intended, a relatively permanent catheter designed by Tenckhoff is used. This tube is placed through a tunnel several inches long in the abdominal wall to reduce the chances that bacteria from the skin will reach the peritoneum through the catheter tract (Fig. 13-5).

Prewarmed sterile dialysate is allowed to flow by gravity into the peritoneal

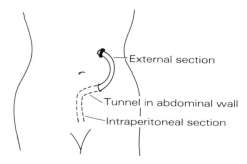

Figure 13-5. Placement of catheter for long-term peritoneal dialysis.

cavity, usually 2 liters at a time. After an equilibration period, the fluid is drained by siphoning and replaced with fresh fluid. The cycle is repeated about every 45 minutes. A dialysis treatment may take from 12 to 36 hours, depending on the needs of the patient. An average patient who is being maintained on long-term peritoneal dialysis may have a 12-hour treatment three times each week. As with hemodialysis, such patients can be trained to carry out the procedure themselves with equipment kept in their own homes.

A more recent refinement of peritoneal dialysis, known as continuous ambulatory peritoneal dialysis (CAPD), allows continuous, around-the-clock peritoneal dialysis. This technique requires changing the dialysate only four or five times every 24 hours. Thus the fluid is allowed to remain in the peritoneal cavity for at least four hours at a time, while the patient goes about his activities. This is a much slower treatment than the intermittent peritoneal dialysis just described, which involves frequent exchanges of fluid. CAPD also uses less total dialysate than intermittent dialysis, but the greater time available for chemical equilibration between blood and fluid seems to make up for this.

Peritoneal dialysis fluid is similar to that used for hemodialysis except in one important respect: the glucose content, which may be 1.5% (1500 mg/dl) to 4.25% (4250 mg/dl) and occasionally even higher. The extra glucose renders the dialysate hypertonic to plasma and causes ultrafiltration of plasma water into the peritoneal cavity, from which it is removed when the dialysis fluid is drained. This is essentially the same process of fluid removal accomplished in hemodialysis by a hydrostatic pressure gradient in the dialyzer. The glucose content of the dialysate is adjusted to the amount of ultrafiltration desired: More hypertonic solution removes more fluid.

Problems Directly Related to Peritoneal Dialysis

Peritonitis and Catheter Infection

A small break in sterile technique when the dialysis catheter is being connected or disconnected can cause bacteria to be introduced into the peritoneal cavity, causing peritonitis. This complication is fairly common in patients with permanent peritoneal catheters, some of whom have frequent episodes of infection. Ordinarily these infections can be treated with continuing dialysis and the addition of antibiotics to the dialysate. Occasionally the infection becomes severe, requiring more drastic measures. Continued or recurrent infections will obstruct the free flow of fluid through the catheter and, with scarring of the peritoneal membrane, may decrease the adequacy of dialysis. In extreme situations repeated infections may make peritoneal dialysis impossible.

Sometimes the skin becomes infected at the exit site of the catheter. This may necessitate removal of the catheter, with subsequent replacement after the infection has been eradicated.

Malfunctions in the Plumbing

For reasons that are sometimes mysterious, peritoneal catheters may fail to function. The usual problem is that fluid that has been placed into the abdominal cavity will not drain out. Perhaps the catheter is in a poor position where it may be partially blocked by abdominal organs. Sometimes it is plugged with fibrin. If function cannot be restored by tinkering with it, the catheter may have to be removed and replaced.

Dialysis fluid has been known to leak out of the peritoneal cavity into preexisting hernias or the abdominal wall or to escape along the catheter tract. If severe and persistent, such difficulties may require discontinuation of peritoneal dialysis.

Mishaps During Catheter Placement

If the operator is unlucky enough to tear a blood vessel, bleeding into the abdominal cavity may be sufficiently severe to require transfusion or to occlude the catheter with clots. Occasionally the bowel is perforated during catheter placement, necessitating surgical exploration and repair. Such accidents are more common in patients with a history of previous surgery, whose viscera may be fixed in place by adhesions.

Hyperglycemia

A significant amount of glucose diffuses from the dialysate into the circulation, especially when solutions with very high glucose concentrations are used. This glucose is easily metabolized by most people, but it can cause severe hyperglycemia in patients with diabetes mellitus. Insulin is sometimes added to the dialysis fluid to promote metabolism of the glucose that is absorbed.

Protein Loss

All patients on peritoneal dialysis lose significant amounts of protein into the dialysate and usually have low serum albumin concentrations, requiring a diet with more protein than is recommended for hemodialysis patients.

PERITONEAL DIALYSIS VERSUS HEMODIALYSIS

In comparison with hemodialysis, peritoneal dialysis has a number of advantages. It takes longer to remove the same amount of fluid and small molecules, but this can be beneficial under some circumstances. Because of this slower, gentler action, peritoneal dialysis is less likely to cause hypotension or disequilibrium and may therefore be preferable in patients with fragile cardiovascular status. The longer period of contact between dialysis fluid and the membrane, especially in the case of CAPD, is theoretically advantageous for the removal of "middle molecules," substances of intermediate molecular weight that may include some uremic toxins. Peritoneal dialysis does not require vascular access or anticoagulation of the patient's blood; this may be an advantage especially in diabetics, who are prone to retinal hemorrhages. The technique of peritoneal dialysis is simpler and easier to learn, so peritoneal dialysis is performed at home by some patients who would not be able to cope with hemodialysis. The paraphernalia are also less formidable than those needed for hemodialysis, especially in the case of CAPD, which requires little equipment except plastic bags of dialysis fluid. This makes it relatively easy for the patient to travel.

With all these advantages of peritoneal dialysis, you may wonder why anyone would choose hemodialysis and why the vast majority of chronic dialysis patients are on hemodialysis. One reason is that chronic hemodialysis has been in widespread use much longer than chronic peritoneal dialysis; this is especially true in the case of CAPD, which is a newcomer to the dialysis scene. Seniority is not the only virtue of hemodialysis, however.

A major advantage of hemodialysis is that it does not require invasion of the peritoneal cavity. Thus the patient on chronic hemodialysis is not exposed to the risk of peritonitis. He does not have a tube penetrating the abdominal wall and (unless he has an external arteriovenous shunt, a rarity these days) can go swimming or engage in other active pursuits with little inhibition. For the patient with a well-functioning internal arteriovenous fistula, or even two such sites for vascular access, hemodialysis is probably a more reliable procedure than peritoneal dialysis, in which plumbing malfunctions have often interrupted treatment. Hemodialysis requires less time on treatment but also more alert supervision during the treatment.

At present, neither system of dialysis emerges as clearly better for everyone. Each technique is superior for certain patients. Many people now on maintenance peritoneal dialysis are refugees from difficult hemodialysis experiences, but hemodialysis programs also support a number of dropouts from peritoneal dialysis. For many patients who would do well with either type of dialysis, the choice is an arbitrary one.

WHO GOES ON DIALYSIS—AND WHEN?

The use of dialysis in the treatment of acute renal failure was discussed in Chapter 11. In this setting dialysis is a temporary holding operation to support the patient until his own kidneys recover.

Most dialysis treatments today are done for chronic renal failure. The symptoms and signs of chronic renal failure, described in the preceding chapter, often creep up on the patient over a period of months or years, making it difficult at times to know when to intervene with dialysis. Sometimes a specific event, such as an episode of pulmonary edema due to fluid retention, will precipitate the decision, but maintenance dialysis often is started simply to ameliorate a constellation of slowly developing uremic symptoms. As a general rule, an adult with a creatinine clearance greater than 10 ml/min can usually be managed without dialysis, whereas a clearance less than 5 ml/min almost guarantees the need for dialysis. For patients who fall between these numbers, the need for dialysis is highly variable. At any level of renal function, though, the most important information affecting this decision is a careful clinical evaluation of the patient. All these medical considerations must be taken into account, as well as social factors (where the patient lives in relation to the dialysis center, family support, etc.) and psychological factors.

In the early days of chronic maintenance hemodialysis, facilities were limited, and only a few patients who were considered most promising were accepted. Usually these were relatively young, productive people without significant medical problems except for renal disease. Though maintenance dialysis is still very costly, public financing and a massive expansion of dialysis facilities have now made it possible to put virtually anyone with advanced renal failure on dialysis. Most physicians will not apply such treatment to persons who are about to die of other causes, such as malignancy, but the chronic dialysis population today includes patients with marginal cardiac or pulmonary function, the myriad complications of advanced diabetes mellitus, and other catastrophic problems. As might be expected, such patients usually do not thrive on dialysis; some of them seem to be existing from one complication to the next. It is difficult to make the decision that a patient's quality of life is too poor to justify continued support, but the need for such judgments may increase in the future as increasing numbers of dialysis candidates put pressure on limited health care resources.

LIFE ON CHRONIC DIALYSIS

By the standards of 30 years ago, dialysis is a miracle. Even so, it is not a complete substitute for normal kidneys. It does not, for instance, replace the hormonal functions of the kidneys, such as production of erythropoietin or $1,25(OH)_2$ vitamin D_3 (calcitriol). Dialysis replaces only the excretory functions of the kidneys, and then only partially; after all, we're trying to replace full-time organs with a part-time treatment. The effectiveness of dialysis could be improved by means of longer treatments, but this would encroach further on the patient's time. Remember also that since dialysis depends on diffusion gradients, its effectiveness decreases as the chemical state of the patient improves; that is, less urea is removed in the fourth hour of dialysis than during the first hour, and even less would be removed per hour thereafter. So a dialysis schedule is a compromise designed to achieve an acceptable chemical state and relief of major uremic symptoms with a tolerable amount of treatment.

This being the case, patients on maintenance dialysis are like people with a moderate degree of chronic renal failure. They may have some of the symptoms and problems described in the last chapter, and they need to observe similar dietary restrictions. Given a constant number of hours of dialysis per week, their blood urea levels will depend largely on their protein intake. In some respects they are more restricted than patients with moderate chronic renal failure, because daily urine volume usually falls sharply after maintenance dialysis is instituted, and with it the output of sodium and potassium. So the intake of water, sodium, and potassium must be limited carefully, or hazardous amounts will accumulate between dialysis treatments. These patients must also continue to take aluminum-containing phosphate binders because phosphate is not usually removed adequately by dialysis.

The anemia that is usual in chronic renal failure may become very severe in dialysis patients, whose problem may be aggravated by losses of blood, iron, and vitamins during treatment. In cases where severe anemia is causing intolerable symptoms and other measures are not effective, periodic blood transfusions may be necessary. Sexual dysfunction, especially impotence, is another major burden for many dialysis patients.

Some patients on maintenance dialysis feel chronically ill; others feel almost normal. Much depends on whether the patient has other medical problems, his state of mind, his ability to observe an appropriate diet, and whether he is receiving an adequate amount of dialysis. The most successful chronic dialysis patients appear to be disciplined people who have learned to accept the necessary restrictions as a part of their lifestyle.

Certain of the difficulties associated with chronic renal failure, such as osteodystrophy, neuropathy, and pericarditis, are fairly common in dialysis patients and are probably seen more often now than they were in predialysis days. Some of these problems take a long time to develop. Their occurrence demonstrates the limitations of dialysis but also reflects its success in keeping people alive long after they would otherwise have died. Indeed, some patients have now been maintained on hemodialysis for 20 years.

BIBLIOGRAPHY

T. Manis and E. A. Friedman. Dialytic therapy for irreversible uremia. *N. Engl. J. Med.* 301: 1260–1265 and 1321–1328, 1979.

D. G. Oreopoulos. Chronic peritoneal dialysis. *Clin. Nephrol.* 9: 165–173, 1978.

R. P. Popovich, J. W. Moncrief, K. D. Nolph, et al. Continuous ambulatory peritoneal dialysis. *Ann. Intern. Med.* 88: 449–456, 1978.

The following articles deal with social, economic, and political aspects of chronic renal failure and its treatment. The first one was written by a patient and his wife.

J. D. Campbell and A. R. Campbell. The social and economic costs of end-stage renal disease. *N. Engl. J. Med.* 299: 386–392, 1978.

E. A. Friedman, B. G. Delano, and K. M. H. Butt. Pragmatic realities in uremia therapy. *N. Engl. J. Med.* 298: 368–371, 1978.

D. S. Greenberg. Renal politics. *N. Engl. J. Med.* 298: 1427–1428, 1978.

S. D. Roberts, D. R. Maxwell, and T. L. Gross. Cost-effective care of end-stage renal disease: A billion dollar question. *Ann. Intern. Med.* 92 (Part 1): 243–248, 1980.

14
Renal Transplantation

In December of 1954, Richard Herrick was a patient in the U.S. Public Health Service Hospital in Boston, and he was in trouble. Richard had chronic renal failure, and his kidney function had gradually deteriorated to the point where he could not hope to live much longer. As we have already seen, chronic dialysis was not yet available. However, unlike most patients in his predicament, Richard was lucky; he had an identical twin, Ronald. By 1954 some preliminary studies had been done in human renal transplantation, although there had been no real successes. In near desperation, Richard was transferred to the Peter Bent Brigham Hospital and received one of his brother's kidneys. No drugs were given to prevent Richard's body from rejecting this kidney because he and his brother were identical twins. Their compatibility was tested before the transplant by means of a skin graft from Ronald to Richard, and no rejection occurred. It was proven again when Richard lived for seven more years, becoming the first long-term success in transplantation. He died because his original kidney disease came back in the transplanted kidney, and Ronald had no more kidneys to give.

The doctors at the Peter Bent Brigham Hospital had been experimenting with renal transplants for a few years before Richard Herrick's historic transplant. These were all transplants from one unrelated person to another, that is, allografts (allo = other, in Greek), and none of them had worked for very long. During the late 1950s the same doctors experimented with total-body irradiation to prevent rejection and, in 1959, performed another twin transplant. This time, however, the twins were not identical. The recipient was given a very small dose of irradiation because it was recognized that large amounts were dangerous. The dose used, however, would now be considered too small to have any significant effect. These twins must have been very similar because the transplant functioned without difficulties for nine months. When signs of rejection appeared at that point, the patient was treated with hydrocortisone injections, and the attack subsided. This may have been the first time corticosteroids were used in treating transplant rejection. Soon after that the immunosuppressive properties of a new compound, azathioprine,

Dr. Michael Madden was a coauthor of this chapter.

were discovered, and in 1962 a transplant was performed from a cadaver donor using a combination of immunosuppressive drugs. Today the combination of prednisone and azathioprine is the most common therapy to prevent rejection.

THE UNDISCRIMINATING WATCHDOG

Rejection is the major obstacle to transplantation of any organ. Lymphocytes in the body are able to recognize and attack cells that are not a part of the body; their vigilance helps to protect us against invaders such as bacteria. But like the watchdog that attacks the postman as well as the prowler, the lymphocytes also attack cells in the transplant because they can detect foreign molecules (antigens) on the cell surfaces. Richard Herrick did not have this problem because his brother's antigens were identical to his, so the lymphocytes could not distinguish his brother's kidney from his own. But, since most transplanted kidneys do not come from identical twins, an assault by the recipient's lymphocytes is almost inevitable.

Various methods have been used to block this attack. The body can be depleted of lymphocytes by draining lymph from the thoracic duct. Or the lymphocytes themselves can be attacked by drugs such as corticosteroids, azathioprine, or an antilymphocyte globulin. Unfortunately, these techniques also diminish the ability to attack invading microorganisms, and thus they make the patient more vulnerable to infection. Research is being done on ways of inducing tolerance, that is, fooling the lymphocytes into accepting the graft as nonforeign; but we don't really know how to do it yet.

One of the best ways to prevent rejection, or at least make it less severe and easier to treat, is to use kidneys whose antigens are as similar as possible to those of the recipient. The closer we come to an identical match, the less aggressive the lymphocytes will be.

FINDING A GOOD TISSUE MATCH

Trying to find a kidney with the right surface antigens for a particular recipient can be difficult and often frustrating. Each person has many different reactive proteins on his cells, representing a small sampling from the great variety of antigens to be found in the human family. Nobody knows definitely how many antigens there are on each cell or in the population pool—and which ones really matter.

We do know positively that the major blood groups of a kidney donor and recipient must be compatible, as they would need to be for a blood transfusion. For instance, a person with group B blood has preformed antibodies against an antigen found on the cells of persons with blood group A. These antibodies would demolish the cells of an A kidney just as they agglutinate

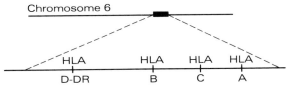

Figure 14-1. Diagram of the region on chromosome 6 that carries the determinants for HLA antigens and MLC reactivity.

group A red blood cells. However, the Rh type of a transplanted kidney does not seem to matter, and the donor and the recipient need not be of the same sex.

Much attention has been focused on the HLA (human leukocyte antigen) system, a group of surface antigens and the genes that code for them. Though most of the research on this system has been done using white blood cells, these antigens are actually found on all nucleated cells in the body and are believed to be important determinants of whether a transplanted tissue will be recognized as foreign or compatible; hence they are sometimes called *histocompatibility antigens.* The chromosome that carries the genes for these proteins contains at least three of them in different places, or loci (Fig. 14-1). These three areas are called HLA loci A, B, and C, and each has its own assortment of possible genes. In a given individual, of course, each locus on the chromosome contains only one of the possible genes for that site. Since chromosomes come in pairs, every person has six loci, three inherited from the father and three from the mother, each coding for a different surface antigen. Some people may have fewer than six of these antigens if the same gene is duplicated in the chromosome pair.

When a kidney becomes available from a cadaver donor, typing of HLA antigens is usually carried out on cells from the donor so that the kidney can be given to someone who shares at least some of the same antigens. (Considering the number of genes in the population, a perfect match would be highly improbable.) It is recognized however, that HLA typing is of limited usefulness (some say it's not useful at all) in predicting transplantation success when cadaver kidneys are involved. Perhaps this is because we have not yet identified all the important determinants of histocompatibility.

If we are dealing with transplantation between siblings, however, the HLA profile tells us more. If the donor and recipient share exactly the same HLA antigens, then they must almost surely have inherited the same pair of chromosomes from their parents. That means they have also inherited in common all of the other genes on those chromosomes, some of which may be important but not identifiable.

One of the other sites on the same chromosome pair that may be quite influential is called HLA-D (Fig. 14-1). The antigens derived from the HLA-D genes are not detected with antibodies (antiserum). Instead we use lymphocytes to reveal them. If we mix the lymphocytes of the patient and those of the donor in a test tube, the lymphocytes after a while will react to each other, unless they are identical at the HLA-D locus. We can then measure the intensity of their proliferative response and compare that to the reaction we would have seen if we had used totally unrelated lymphocytes in the test tube. If there is no reaction (HLA-D identity), we call that 0% MLC (*mixed lymphocyte culture*) reactivity. If the recipient's lymphocytes react as much to the donor's lymphocytes as they do to totally unrelated cells, that is 100% reactivity, and the chances for rejection are far greater.

The mixed lymphocyte culture is a useful test, but it requires seven days and is therefore not helpful where we need it most—in cadaver-kidney transplantation—since we can't keep the kidney viable that long. A solution to this problem may be to measure DR (D-related) antigens, which are closely identified with the D locus and can be detected fairly quickly with antiserum. There is still controversy about whether testing for DR antigens is actually measuring the important D locus or whether there is a separate DR locus.

The final test needed before performing transplantation is a cross-match, which detects preformed antibodies against surface antigens. This is similar to the procedure used to check a blood transfusion before giving it. The cells of the donor (lymphocytes again) are mixed with the serum of the patient in the presence of rabbit complement. If the cells are killed, the cross-match is positive, and the kidney would be rejected in an accelerated fashion if it were transplanted to that recipient. There are quite a few patients awaiting transplantation who have little chance of getting a kidney because they have preformed antibodies against a large number of human surface antigens.

FINDING KIDNEYS TO TRANSPLANT

There are basically two sources of kidneys for transplantation: live relatives and cadavers. A significant minority of patients have a healthy close relative whose kidney matches their own tissues well enough to offer a good chance of avoiding rejection. Usually that means a brother or sister, occasionally a parent or a child. (Parent-to-child or child-to-parent transplants are usually not HLA-identical, because the child got half of his genes from the other parent). Obviously we try very hard to be sure that a living related donor is a close match, and we don't use poor matches. Even though the donor can live perfectly well with only one remaining kidney, it does not seem justifiable to put a healthy person through the risks and stresses of major surgery if the chances of success are not very good.

A well-matched living-donor transplant, however, is miles ahead of most cadaver-donor transplants. It is very hard to find a cadaver kidney that is nearly as good a match as a relative's kidney can be. For that reason, living-donor transplant patients can often get along with less immunosuppressive medication (prednisone and azathioprine), and they have a much higher rate of success. There are exceptions, of course. Every large transplantation program has had some failures with living-donor kidneys and excellent results with many cadaver kidneys. Sometimes the same patient has done well with a cadaver graft after rejecting the kidney of a relative. Obviously, tissue matching is not yet an exact science.

Where does a cadaver kidney come from, and how is it retrieved without damaging it? Cadaver kidneys are taken from the victims of automobile accidents and other conditions that destroy the brain without harming the kidneys. The ideal donor is a young person with no prior medical problems whose organs are likely to be healthy. The kidneys need to be removed very carefully to avoid trauma. Ideally this should be done while the heart of the donor is still beating, though that can create ethical or legal problems. Whatever the approach, the kidneys will be permanently damaged if they remain at body or room temperature without circulation for very long. If a person is killed on the highway and brought to the hospital 45 minutes later, it is already too late to use his kidneys.

Cadaver kidneys cannot be stored indefinitely. The length of time between their removal and transplantation depends upon the method of storage, whether on ice or in a special perfusion machine, but generally they must be used within two or three days, and the sooner the better. Even with such treatment, cadaver kidneys sometimes fail to function for about 10 days after they are transplanted because of reversible damage that resembles acute tubular necrosis.

Though many problems remain to be solved, renal transplantation is no longer an experimental procedure. It has brought a new life to many people, and about 2500 kidney transplants are performed every year in the United States alone. It is also estimated, however, that approximately 7500 patients are waiting on dialysis to receive a kidney. Some of them wait only a few days or weeks, but most of them will have to wait for months or even years until a suitably matched kidney becomes available. Considering the number of accidental deaths every year, much of this delay should not be necessary. Unfortunately, many good kidneys get buried in cemeteries with their original owners because doctors, nurses, and relatives of accident victims are not aware of the need for them.

THOSE WHO WAIT

Who are all these people waiting to get cadaver kidneys? How does a person with kidney disease get on that list?

When transplantation first started, it was very selective. Only the healthiest patients were even considered, that is, those with no evidence of other serious diseases (especially coronary artery disease, ulcer disease, or obstructive lung disease) and no systemic disease such as diabetes mellitus. The criteria for transplantation have enlarged considerably, however, and now many more patients are considered candidates. Many transplant centers work on the motto: "If you can be dialyzed, you can get a transplant." Realistically, however, there are some limits. For example, no one would transplant a kidney to a patient who was expected to die soon of some other problem, such as an uncontrollable malignancy.

There are many other conditions that do not immediately eliminate a patient from consideration but do increase the risks associated with transplantation. One of these conditions is age. Most centers prefer not to accept patients who are more than 55 years old. Beyond that age the risks of surgery increase, and the chances of success diminish. This limit is not an absolute one, however, and the individual patient's wishes sometimes go a long way in making this decision.

Patients with severe coronary disease or pulmonary disease have an especially difficult time convincing the surgeon to operate. Their risk is much greater than that of otherwise healthy dialysis patients. The overall risks are also greater for a person with diabetes mellitus. These patients frequently have serious vascular disease, and they are much more susceptible to severe infections. This makes it rather risky to give them immunosuppressive drugs. For these reasons diabetics were excluded from transplant lists for many years and even today are accepted with some foreboding. Many have done quite well following transplantation, however, and this may be the treatment of choice for young diabetics with renal failure, especially since they often have more than their share of problems on chronic dialysis.

The distinction between a living-related and a cadaver graft may occasionally make the decision for or against a transplant. A marginal patient is a better risk if he is to get a related kidney. On the other hand, a surgeon may be reluctant to take a kidney from a relative if the patient himself is so great a risk that his survival is questionable. Obviously the decision is not an easy one.

WHEN THE TELEPHONE RINGS

Living-donor transplants are scheduled in advance and performed during convenient daylight hours. But the patient who is on the waiting list for a cadaver kidney is essentially on 24-hour call to the hospital; one never knows when a kidney will become available.

When the call comes, the recipient hurries to the hospital, where a final cross-match is done. Surgery is then performed as soon as possible. A kidney graft is generally placed in the pelvis, in the retroperitoneal space, with the iliac artery and vein used for its blood supply. The new ureter is implanted into the patient's own bladder. Most patients still have their own kidneys emptying into the bladder also, since their native kidneys are not removed unless necessitated by severe hypertension or recurrent infection. Sometimes this makes it difficult to tell immediately after the operation how well the new kidney is working just by watching the urine flow. Eventually the serum creatinine usually begins to decrease, the urine flow increases, and the operation is at least a temporary success. If problems arise with the new kidney, its relatively superficial position in the pelvis makes it easier to investigate the trouble.

Several days after the operation the kidney may not yet be working. It may still be recovering from the acute tubular necrosis that developed during removal and storage. Of course, it could be suffering early rejection or any of a number of technical problems, such as obstruction of the new artery, vein, or ureter. These possibilities also have to be considered, even after the patient returns home, whenever there is a decrease in the function of the kidneys. Sometimes the original disease that caused the first set of kidneys to fail will return. This is what happened to Richard Herrick, and it is a concern in many transplants, especially in those patients who originally had certain forms of glomerulonephritis.

Usually, however, when the transplant patient suffers a decrease in kidney function, rejection is the culprit. There are few transplant recipients who have not experienced at least one or two mild episodes. Rejection may take several forms that differ in their mechanisms of damage and the interval following transplantation in which they usually occur.

A *hyperacute* or *accelerated rejection,* which occurs immediately or within days, is a violent reaction caused by circulating antibodies that destroy the kidney promptly regardless of any treatment employed. Usually it can be avoided by means of the preoperative cross-match. *Acute rejection,* which usually begins in the first few weeks, is mediated by lymphocytes. Unless very severe, it often responds favorably to an increase in the dose of corticosteroids and may or may not happen again when the dose is decreased. *Chronic rejection* tends to occur later than the other forms of rejection. It is probably caused by antibodies and attacks the blood vessels of the kidney graft. No treatment seems to be effective. A biopsy of the transplanted kidney sometimes helps to distinguish between the various forms of rejection and other problems.

Chronic rejection is a slowly progressing disease, and the patient who is gradually losing his transplanted kidney can be managed like those with worsening end-stage renal disease. Depending on their overall status, these patients are usually offered the same options of chronic dialysis or another transplant that were offered them when they first were found to have severe chronic kidney disease. There are many patients who have had two or more transplanted kidneys, each of which may have worked adequately for several years. These patients must be considered at least partial successes in that they were spared the stresses of repeated dialysis treatments for at least a few years.

CALCULATING THE ODDS—AND THE RISKS

Figure 14-2 summarizes the chances of success with living-related and cadaver grafts. If we compare the results two years after surgery, we find that

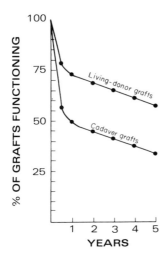

Figure 14-2. Functional survival of kidney grafts from living related donors and cadaver donors. These data come from the last (1977) report of the Human Renal Transplant Registry. The subgroup of living-donor grafts from HLA-identical siblings has a substantially higher success rate than that reflected in this figure, which shows the results of all grafts from living donors regardless of match. Survival of recipients is better than that of their grafts, since most patients return to dialysis following transplant failure.

about 70% of kidneys from relatives and 45% of kidneys from cadavers are still supporting their new owners. You will note that the kidney-survival curves become straighter with the passage of time; that is, the rate of failure is decreased after the first two years, so the person whose kidney is working well at that point has a good chance that it will continue to function for many more years. How long can it last? No one knows, but many patients are now into their second decade with a transplanted kidney. Most of these long-term success stories involve well-matched kidneys from relatives, but some people with cadaver kidneys are also in this group.

Though only half of the cadaver grafts are still functioning after two years, the survival of the patients who received them is considerably better than that. Still, there is a significant mortality associated with renal transplantation. Any major operation entails cardiac and pulmonary risks, of course, but most of the patients who die soon after transplantation succumb to severe infection. This hazard is related to the large doses of immunosuppressive drugs that they must receive in the postoperative period to block graft rejection. Unfortunately, these agents also inhibit the body's response to infection, and transplant recipients are sometimes overwhelmed by agents, such as cytomegalovirus, that do not cause problems in people with normal immune systems. Survival has improved over the last several years, however, as more centers have abandoned the attitude that the kidney must be saved at all costs. Obviously it does not make sense to kill the recipient with high doses of immunosuppressive drugs while trying to save the graft. If he loses his transplanted kidney, the patient can always go back to dialysis and wait for another kidney that may be a better match.

Infection is not the only side effect of treatment with corticosteroids. The entire spectrum of Cushing's syndrome may be seen, especially changes in the body habitus (moon facies, centripetal fat distribution, etc.). Other, more serious problems include cataracts, osteoporosis, aseptic necrosis of the hip joints, fragile skin and easy bruisability, and development or worsening of diabetes mellitus. These effects can be truly disabling, but they can be avoided in large part by using smaller doses of steroids. Many patients can be maintained on almost insignificant doses of these drugs after the first year, but this is often not possible in those with cadaver kidneys.

TRANSPLANTATION VERSUS DIALYSIS

There is no denying the fact that transplantation today is still a gamble. We know that some patients will be winners and others losers, but the outcome for any given patient cannot be assured in advance. The odds of being a winner are considerably better in renal transplantation than in the halls of Las Vegas or Monte Carlo, but the stakes in transplantation—health or even one's life—would make many veteran casino gamblers turn pale.

Patients whose kidney transplants are successful are no longer bound to the dialysis machine and its demands on their time. Their graft restores all the endocrine functions of the kidney and maintains a normal chemical environment without the need for dietary restrictions. Dialysis can never do all that. Because of the improved chemical environment, complications of renal failure such as osteodystrophy or neuropathy may be arrested or reversed. Since these patients in general feel better, they are more likely to return to their jobs and other normal activities. Although transplantation is expensive, it costs less in the long run than repetitive dialysis.

Those who are less fortunate may require substantial doses of corticosteroids for long periods of time to protect a poorly functioning graft their body is trying to reject; they have traded total renal failure for the side effects of steroids with partial renal failure. The most obvious losers are those whose grafts are rejected within the first few weeks. After more than a month of debilitating hospitalization, often complicated by infection, they leave the hospital without their new kidneys—and sometimes they do not leave alive.

Which patients should take the gamble of transplantation? The decision must be made on an individual basis, but certain factors will influence it heavily. The availability of a well-matched kidney from a healthy relative makes transplantation more attractive because the odds for success are better. For those who are doing poorly on dialysis—developing neuropathy or osteodystrophy or just not feeling well—it may be easier to accept the risks of transplantation. This reasoning often applies to diabetics, whose vision may also be deteriorating. Many patients chafe under the dietary restrictions and constraints on their freedom that go with dialysis. Young people especially often feel that such limitations make it impossible for them to lead a normal life; since they are also better surgical risks, transplantation is a good choice for many of them.

Other patients—especially older, settled people—can accept the restrictions of dialysis more easily. For them surgery would be more hazardous and the chances of success less. If their condition remains satisfactory and they feel well enough to do what they want to do, why should they gamble on transplantation?

A final word of caution is in order: Survival figures published by various dialysis and transplantation centers are virtually worthless for a comparison between these two methods of treatment. The reason is that patients are not assigned to treatment on a random basis; they are selected according to certain criteria, and this means that one program may have patients who were better risks initially than those in another program. In the absence of valid comparative data, it seems reasonable to assume that neither form of therapy is clearly superior and that each patient must be matched with the treatment that best fits his situation.

BIBLIOGRAPHY

F. H. Bach and J. J. van Rood. The major histocompatibility complex—genetics and biology. *N. Engl. J. Med.* 295: 806–813, 872–878, 929–936, 1976.

A fairly detailed review of basic knowledge about the factors determining histocompatibility.

C. B. Carpenter. HLA and renal transplantation. *N. Engl. J. Med.* 302: 860–862, 1980.

Summarizes current knowledge about histocompatibility and transplantation.

W. A. Check. New approaches to prolonging survival of transplanted organs. *J.A.M.A.* 242: 2265–2273, 1979.

Lively account of diverse efforts to beat the rejection problem.

R. A. Guttman. Renal transplantation. *N. Engl. J. Med.* 301: 975–982 and 1038–1048, 1979.

General survey of current thinking and practice.

The Surgical Clinics of North America, Vol. 58, No. 2, April 1978.

A symposium on organ transplantation appears in this issue. Included are a number of articles on kidney transplantation and closely related subjects.

Glossary of Renal and Related Terms

During his childhood, one of the authors tried to learn something about sex by looking into a medical book. The attempt was futile; even the simplest mechanics of the process were camouflaged by incomprehensible medical terminology. In an effort to protect our readers against similar frustrations, we offer the following glossary of some important terms used in this book.

Limitations of space dictate that not all terms used in the book can be defined in the glossary. Some words are used infrequently and may be explained where they appear. Many anatomical terms describing parts of the kidney or the nephron are defined in Chapter 2, and the special vocabulary used to describe lesions in the glomeruli is explained in Chapter 9. When a term does not appear in the glossary, the index may help you to locate an explanation in the text. Usually we have not attempted to define words that are a common part of medical-biological vocabulary (e.g., hematocrit, leukocytosis, neuropathy); the reader should refer to a general medical dictionary if any of these are unfamiliar.

Many of the subjects that appear in the glossary are defined or discussed at some length in the text. Rather than repeat the whole explanation in the glossary, we refer the reader to the appropriate pages or chapter.

Acidosis. A state of abnormal hydrogen-ion accumulation in the body as reflected by arterial pH below 7.35.

Active Transport. The movement of a substance across a barrier, such as a biologic membrane, against a physical-chemical gradient. Active transport therefore requires the expenditure of energy.

Aldosterone. The naturally occurring mineralocorticoid hormone in man; its major effect on the kidney is to promote sodium resorption and potassium excretion. Discussed on page 64.

Alkalosis. A state of low hydrogen-ion concentration in the body as reflected by arterial pH above 7.45.

Allograft. A tissue graft taken from a donor who is of the same species as the recipient but of different genetic composition (i.e., not an identical twin).

Alternative Pathway of complement activation. A chemical sequence that results in stimulation of C3 and later-acting components of the complement system without prior activation of C1, C4, and C2. See also **Complement.**

Aminoaciduria. The presence of amino acids in the urine in excess of the minute quantities that may be present normally.

Angiotensin. See **Renin-angiotensin system.**

Anion Gap. Defined and discussed on pages 110–112.

Antidiuretic hormone (ADH) (also known as *vasopressin*). A peptide hormone that acts to increase resorption of water by the kidneys, thus decreasing the volume and increasing the osmolality of the urine. Explained more fully on pages 50–51. Its action on the kidneys is described on page 79.

Autoregulation of glomerular filtration rate and renal blood flow. A mechanism, apparently intrinsic in the kidney, that allows glomerular filtration rate and renal blood flow to remain relatively constant despite changes in systemic blood pressure. Described and discussed on pages 19–21.

Azotemia. An abnormally high concentration of nitrogenous waste products in the blood, such as is found in renal failure. Strictly speaking, this word refers only to a chemical state, while the term *uremia* denotes the symptoms and clinical illness (described in Chapter 12) associated with severe renal failure.

Calcitriol. 1,25 Dihydroxycholecalciferol, believed to be the active form of vitamin D (see page 201).

Casts. Microscopic cylindrical structures that may be found in the urine. Formed in the renal tubules, casts consist of a protein matrix in which cells may or may not be embedded (see page 128). They often provide information about the presence of renal disease and its type, though hyaline casts may be formed at times in normal kidneys.

Cholecalciferol. The chemical name of vitamin D_3.

Clearance. Renal clearance is an expression of the efficiency with which the kidneys remove a substance from the plasma. The clearance is the number of milliliters of plasma needed each minute to supply the amount of the substance being excreted in the urine per minute. One may think of it as the number of milliliters of plasma that are being cleared of the substance each minute, though the "cleared" plasma cannot be identified because of constant mixing with other plasma. Though usually expressed as milliliters per minute, clearance is also expressed sometimes as liters per day.

A clearance measurement relates the renal elimination of a substance to its plasma level. Thus it compensates automatically for the fact that some substances are excreted in greater absolute amounts when their plasma levels are high, even though renal function is unchanged. The clearance concept is developed in Chapter 3, especially on pages 29–32.

Complement.   A complex system of plasma proteins that interact in cascades and amplify the effects of many antigen-antibody reactions. There are two recognized pathways of complement activation, known as the *classical pathway* and the *alternative pathway.* Activation of the classical pathway usually requires an antigen-antibody reaction involving either immunoglobulins G (IgG) or M (IgM) and complement components C1–C9. Complement may be partially responsible for immune-mediated renal injury. See also **Alternative pathway.**

Countercurrent Exchanger.   An arrangement for passive exchange of material or heat between two streams flowing past each other in opposite directions. As used in renal physiology, this term applies to the diffusion of solutes and water between the ascending and descending portions of the vasa recta as these vessels pass into and out of the hypertonic renal medulla (see page 80). This design decreases the rate at which high solute concentrations in the medulla are dissipated by blood flowing through it.

Countercurrent Hypothesis (countercurrent mechanism).   The explanation now accepted for the basic mechanism of urine concentration in mammalian kidneys. The name derives from the fact that tubular fluid flows in opposite directions in the descending and ascending limbs of Henle's loop and that the operation of the system depends on this feature, as explained on pages 76–84.

Countercurrent Multiplier.   A system in which the ability of a single cell to create an osmotic gradient (the "single effect") is multiplied many times by means of a countercurrent design. The loop of Henle is a countercurrent multiplier.

Deciliter (dl).   0.1 liter; 100 ml.

Diabetes Insipidus.   A disorder characterized by the production of very large volumes of dilute urine. It is caused either by lack of antidiuretic hormone or by failure of the renal tubules to respond to ADH. Discussed on pages 84–85.

Dialysis.   The passive transfer of water and small molecules across a semipermeable membrane in response to differences in their concentrations. A *dialyzer* is an apparatus in which this process takes place, and the *dialysate* is the solution placed on one side of the membrane.

Hemodialysis and *peritoneal dialysis* are methods of applying the principles of dialysis to the treatment of patients with renal failure. Chapter 13 describes dialysis and its clinical applications.

Diuresis.   A greater than usual rate of urine production. A diuresis may be a normal response to a large fluid intake, a response to drugs or osmotic agents, or a disposal of abnormal quantities of fluid previously accumulated in the body. *Diuretic drugs* (or simply *diuretics*) are agents that cause diuresis; those used most commonly act by inhibiting the resorption of sodium or chloride in the renal tubules.

Donnan Effect (also called the *Gibbs-Donnan effect* by some authors).   An unequal distribution of diffusible electrolytes across a membrane at equilibrium, which results from the presence of nondiffusible ions such as proteins. Described and discussed on pages 6–7.

Edema.   An abnormal accumulation in body tissues of interstitial fluid that is sufficient in amount to be seen or felt. Discussed on pages 52–57.

Electron Microscope.   A microscope that utilizes a beam of electrons (rather than a beam of visible light) to form enlarged images of a structure. The shorter wavelengths available with electrons permit much greater magnifications than are possible using light microscopy. *Electron micrographs* are pictures made with the use of an electron microscope. *Electron-dense* structures are those that impede the passage of electrons and are represented as dark areas on transmission electron micrographs. *Scanning electron microscopy* is a technique that uses an electron beam to make highly enlarged pictures of three-dimensional structures (such as an entire unsectioned glomerulus).

Excretory Urogram.   See Intravenous pyelogram.

Extracellular Fluid (ECF, extracellular water).   One of the major body fluid compartments; by strict definition, all of the body water not within cells. Described on pages 2–3. The general role of the ECF as the internal environment of the body is described on pages 41–42.

Fanconi Syndrome.   This name has been applied to a number of disorders. As used in this book, it refers to a dysfunction of proximal tubular cells affecting at least several resorptive transport systems. Substances that may appear in the urine in abnormal amounts include glucose, amino acids, phosphate, and urate.

Filtered Load.   The total amount of a substance that glomerular filtration delivers (per unit of time) to the tubules. This is calculated by multiplying the glomerular filtration rate (usually expressed as ml/min) by the concentration of the substance in glomerular filtrate (mg, mmole, or mEq per ml). The concentration in glomerular filtrate depends on the concentration of the substance in plasma water, its glomerular permeability, binding to plasma proteins, and the Donnan effect in the case of electrolytes. Filtered load is expressed as mass (mg, mmole, or mEq) per minute.

Filtration Fraction.   That fraction of the effective renal plasma flow per minute which is filtered by the glomeruli. Thus the inulin clearance divided by the clearance of para-aminohippurate is equal to the filtration fraction, which in man is usually 16 to 20%.

Fluorescent Antibodies.   Antibodies directed against specific biological substances (often certain proteins) and conjugated with a fluorescent dye. When exposed to biological materials, the antibodies bind to their target antigens. The site of the antigen can then be identified because the dye conjugated to the antibody is fluorescent when exposed to ultraviolet light. For instance, fluorescent antibodies against immunoglobulin G (IgG) can be used to demonstrate the presence and location of IgG that becomes deposited in glomeruli in some renal diseases.

Fractional Excretion.   The fractional excretion of a substance is that fraction of the filtered load that is excreted in the urine.

Glomerulotubular Balance.   The phenomenon by which the proximal tubular resorption of sodium and water appears to adjust to changes in glomerular filtration rate so that a relatively constant fraction of the filtrate is reabsorbed in the proximal tubule and a relatively constant fraction is delivered to more distal parts of the tubule. This is described in more detail on pages 62–63.

Note that glomerulotubular balance applies only to the proximal tubular response to changes in GFR in the absence of other significant physiological changes. When certain other factors are operative, such as expansion of the extracellular fluid volume, changes do occur in the percentage of glomerular filtrate that is reabsorbed in the proximal tubule.

Glomerular Filtration Rate (GFR).   The rate at which plasma water is filtered into Bowman's capsule by all of an individual's glomeruli combined. Described on page 19. Methods of measuring GFR are described on pages 29–32.

Glucosuria (also called *glycosuria*).   The presence of glucose in the urine in excess of the minute amount that may be present normally.

Hematuria.   The presence of red blood cells in the urine.

Hydronephrosis.   Dilatation of the pelvis and calyces of one or both kidneys with urine. Hydronephrosis is usually caused by partial or complete obstruction to the outflow of urine.

Note: The following four terms and their antonyms are defined by reference to normal plasma values. Small variations in these normal values are common among different laboratories. The actual measurements are usually made on serum rather than on plasma.

Hypercalcemia.   A state in which plasma calcium concentration is above the normal range of 8.5 to 10.5 mg/dl (2.1 to 2.6 mmole/liter). *Hypocalcemia* is a state of subnormal plasma calcium concentration.

Hyperkalemia. A state in which plasma potassium concentration is above the normal range of 3.5 to 5.0 mEq/liter (or mmole/liter). *Hypokalemia* is a state of subnormal plasma potassium concentration.

Hypernatremia. A state in which plasma sodium concentration is above the normal range of 135 to 145 mEq/liter (or mmole/liter). *Hyponatremia* is a state of subnormal sodium concentration.

Hyperosmotic (hypertonic). As used in this book, having an osmolality greater than the usual osmolality of plasma (285 to 295 mOsm/kg of water). Hyperosmotic urine is said to be *concentrated.* A *hypo-osmotic* or *hypotonic* solution has an osmolality below that of plasma. Hypo-osmotic urine is also described as *dilute.*

Hypocomplementemia. A state in which the plasma concentration of complement is abnormally low. Though many different proteins comprise the complement system, measurements are made most commonly of C3, C4, or "total hemolytic complement"; the last reflects the overall integrity of the complement system. In practice, therefore, *hypocomplementemia* often refers to low levels of C3, C4, and/or total hemolytic complement.

Immune Complex. An aggregation formed by the binding of a molecule or molecules of antibody to a molecule or molecules of specific antigen. An *immune-complex disease* is one that is believed to be caused by immune complexes.

Immunofluorescence Microscopy. The microscopic examination, using ultraviolet light, of tissues that have been exposed to fluorescent antibodies. Fluorescence identifies the location of the antibodies and the antigens against which they are directed. See also **Fluorescent antibodies.**

Immunosuppressive Drugs. Agents believed to block or reduce the activity of the immune system. Among the drugs most commonly used for this purpose are prednisone (a synthetic analogue of cortisone), azathioprine, and cyclophosphamide. These and other immunosuppressive drugs may be quite different from each other in their mechanisms of action.

Intact Nephron Hypothesis. The proposal that the nephrons contributing to the performance of a chronically diseased kidney are functionally intact. This concept and some of the evidence for it are described on pages 187–189.

Interstitium. A tissue space between other structures. The *renal interstitium* surrounds and lies between the glomeruli, tubules, and blood vessels within the kidney. *Interstitial nephritis*, described more fully on pages 163–166, is a term applied to a group of renal diseases that appear to involve the interstitium primarily. *Interstitial fluid* (page 2) is a part of the extracellular fluid that is found between blood vessels and cells.

Intracellular Fluid (intracellular water). The largest body fluid compartment, consisting of the water within cells. Described on pages 1–2.

Intravenous Pyelogram (IVP), also called *excretory urogram.*   An x-ray study of the upper urinary collecting system. Before the roentgenograms are taken, the patient receives an intravenous injection of an iodine-containing contrast substance that will be excreted by the kidneys. X-ray pictures are taken within one minute following the injection and at timed intervals thereafter. The renal calyces and pelvis and the ureters are delineated by the dense contrast material that passes through them, and the procedure is used primarily to study these structures. Roentgenograms taken during the early part of the study usually show an outline of the kidney tissue also as the iodinated material enters the tubules. Later films outline the bladder. If renal function is severely impaired, the contrast material may be excreted too slowly or concentrated too poorly to provide adequate visualization of the structures.

Inulin.   A polysaccharide, derived from artichokes or dahlia tubers, that is the standard of reference for the measurement of glomerular filtration rate. (*Inulin clearance* equals the GFR.) The characteristics of inulin and its usefulness in the study of renal function are described on pages 29–31.

Isohydric Principle.   A law of chemistry which states that all buffer combinations in the same solution must be in equilibrium with the ambient pH and therefore with each other.

Isosmotic (isotonic).   Having the same osmolality. Thus two fluids of equal osmolality are said to be isosmotic or isotonic. When a solution is said to be isotonic without mention of any other solution, the implied reference solution is usually normal plasma. So an *isotonic saline solution* usually means a solution of sodium chloride having roughly the same osmolality as plasma.

Kallikrein-Kinin System.   Kallikrein is an enzyme that liberates kinins from protein precursors (called kininogens). The kinins are a group of peptide hormones. The best known of these, bradykinin, causes arteriolar dilatation and increased capillary permeability among other effects.

Micropuncture.   The technique of placing a micropipette into the lumen of a minute structure. The most common use of micropuncture in renal physiology has been to enter the lumen of the tubule at some accessible point, such as a superficial loop of proximal tubule. The pipette may be used to obtain tubular fluid for analysis, to measure pressure or electrical potential within the lumen, or to perfuse solutions into the tubule.

Middle Molecules.   Molecules that are intermediate in size between small, easily dialyzed molecules (such as urea) and those that are much too large to be dialyzed (such as proteins). Some investigators believe that accumulation of certain poorly dialyzable middle molecules causes toxic effects in patients with renal failure, including those who are being supported by dialysis.

Milliosmole (mOsm).   0.001 osmole. Explained in some detail on pages 8–9.

Mineralocorticoid Hormones.   A group of steroid hormones produced in the adrenal cortex. Mineralocorticoid hormones exert their major effects on the transport of sodium and potassium (in contrast to the closely related glucocorticoid hormones, which affect glucose metabolism and inhibit inflammatory reactions). See also **Aldosterone.**

Mixed Lymphocyte Culture (MLC).   A laboratory method used to assess the compatibility of a prospective tissue donor and the prospective recipient. The test, which is done by incubating recipient lymphocytes with donor lymphocytes, is described on page 228.

Natriuretic Hormone (natriuretic factor).   A substance that may be produced somewhere in the body in response to expansion of the extracellular fluid volume and that may act on the renal tubules to inhibit the reabsorption of sodium. The existence of such a hormone is controversial at present. See the discussion on pages 69–71.

Nephrolithiasis.   The presence of kidney stones.

Nephrosis, Nephrotic, Nephrotic Syndrome.   These terms refer to a group of glomerular diseases characterized by the loss of large amounts of protein (primarily albumin) in the urine. Any of these diseases may be referred to as *nephrosis.* Heavy proteinuria is often accompanied by edema, a low concentration of plasma albumin, and sometimes elevated levels of blood lipids. Patients who have some of these findings (in addition to proteinuria) are said to have the *nephrotic syndrome,* though some authors use this term when only heavy proteinuria is present. (See discussion on page 128.) *Nephrotic* refers to any disease in this group, to the patient who has such a disease, or to the associated clinical picture. Urine that contains much albumin, sometimes with fat bodies and cholesterol crystals but with few red cells or inflammatory cells, is said to demonstrate a *nephrotic pattern.*

Nephritis, Nephritic.   Strictly speaking, *nephritis* means inflammation of the kidney. When the inflammation is primarily in the glomeruli (glomerulonephritis), the clinical picture is typically characterized by hypertension, edema, and sometimes decreased glomerular filtration, while the urine contains red blood cells and sometimes red-cell casts. The clinical picture of the patient may be described as *nephritic,* and the urinary abnormalities just mentioned represent a *nephritic pattern* (in contrast to the nephrotic pattern). Unfortunately, the term *nephritis* has also been applied to a number of renal diseases that do not appear to have a major inflammatory component, such as membranous glomerulonephritis and focal sclerosing glomerulonephritis. This is confusing.

Nephrotoxic.   Injurious to the kidneys.

Nonionic Diffusion.   This term refers to a process in which the un-ionized, lipid-soluble form of a molecule diffuses easily through cell membranes, in contrast to its ionized, poorly diffusible form. Nonionic diffusion is believed to account for the concentration of NH_4^+ in acid urine, as explained on pages 98–99.

Oliguria.   An abnormally low rate of urine flow. Given the concentrating limits of normal kidneys, each individual needs to produce a certain minimum volume of urine each day in order to excrete his osmolar load. Oliguria could be defined physiologically as urine production below this minimum volume, which would vary for different individuals. For an average-sized adult on an average diet, a urine flow less than 500 ml/day usually constitutes oliguria.

Oncotic Pressure.   The osmotic force exerted by proteins in solution.

Osmole, Osmolality, Osmolarity, Osmotic Pressure or Force.   Explained on pages 7–9.

Osmolar Load (osmotic load).   In renal physiology the total number of solute particles (expressed as milliosmoles) being excreted by the kidneys per unit of time.

Osmotic Diuresis.   An unusually high rate of urine production caused by the presence in the tubules of a large osmolar load. Although most diuretics increase the osmolar load in the tubules, the term *osmotic diuretic* usually refers to agents that add to the body a significant number of new molecules that will be excreted by the kidneys. Mannitol, which is filtered into the tubular system but not reabsorbed, is a good example of an osmotic diuretic. Its action is described briefly on pages 87–88.

Para-Aminohippurate (PAH).   A compound that, after infusion into the circulation, is excreted into the urine by glomerular filtration and tubular secretion. Its efficient removal by the tubular cells makes it possible to use the clearance of PAH as a measure of renal plasma flow, as explained on pages 37–39. It has been employed widely for this purpose by renal physiologists.

PAS Stain (periodic acid-Schiff).   A histochemical staining procedure that is used to identify glycogen, neutral polysaccharides, and glycoproteins.

Plasmapheresis.   The removal of plasma from a subject without significant removal of the cellular elements of the blood; it is usually carried out with the use of a specially designed centrifuge that separates plasma from cells continuously, returning the cells to the patient. The volume of plasma removed is replaced with electrolyte solutions or with albumin or plasma from normal donors. Plasmapheresis has been advocated for the treatment of some renal diseases in which abnormal substances in the plasma (such as antibodies, immune complexes, or macroglobulins) are believed to be responsible for progressive kidney damage. Its effectiveness in such situations is still being evaluated.

Plasma Water.   A part of the extracellular fluid (page 2); the water in which blood cells and platelets are suspended and in which plasma solutes and proteins are dissolved.

Polydipsia.   The ingestion of water or other beverages in unusually large amounts, typically because of excessive thirst.

Polyuria.   The production of an unusually large volume of urine.

Properdin.   A plasma protein involved in activation of complement by the alternative pathway. It is deposited in glomeruli in some forms of glomerulonephritis.

Prostaglandins.   A family of potent hormones derived from arachidonic acid, an unsaturated essential fatty acid. Different prostaglandins appear to have a variety of effects in many organs. In the kidneys prostaglandins may modulate renal blood flow and influence water excretion and renin production, but there are still many unanswered questions about their physiological role.

Proteinuria.   The presence of abnormal quantities of protein in the urine. (Normal adults may excrete up to about 150 mg/day of protein in their urine.) Since albumin is the predominant urinary protein in most renal diseases, the term *albuminuria* is sometimes used instead of *proteinuria,* even though the nonspecific tests usually used show only that some kind of protein is present. The significance of proteinuria is discussed in Chapter 9.

Pyelonephritis.   Renal disease resulting from bacterial infection of the kidney and its pelvis. *Acute pyelonephritis* is an inflammatory process caused by active bacterial infection. *Chronic pyelonephritis* refers to a pattern of morphologic changes in the kidney believed to result from long-standing infection. Considerable confusion has arisen from the fact that such changes may also result from other conditions and thus do not always reflect antecedent infection.

Pyuria.   The occurrence of abnormal numbers of leukocytes in the urine. The finding of pyuria suggests, but does not prove, the presence of infection somewhere in the urinary tract.

Rejection.   A potentially destructive reaction against a tissue graft caused by immunologic mechanisms. The different forms rejection may take in transplanted kidneys are described on page 231.

Renal Blood Flow (RBF).   The total volume of blood flowing per unit of time through both kidneys. *Renal plasma flow* (RPF) is the volume of plasma perfusing both kidneys per unit of time. As explained on pages 37–39, RPF can be measured indirectly by means of the PAH clearance, and RBF can be calculated from the same measurement. Renal plasma flow is about 650 ml/min in an average-sized normal man.

Renal Osteodystrophy.   A disorder of the skeleton that may occur in patients with chronic renal failure. Its causes and manifestations are described on pages 200–202.

Renal Tubular Acidosis (RTA).   Acidosis resulting from failure of individual renal tubules to secrete adequate H^+ (in contrast to acidosis that results from a large reduction in functioning renal tissue). RTA encompasses more than one disorder; its different forms are described on pages 108–110.

Renin-Angiotensin System.   A hormonal system that plays a part in the regulation of blood pressure and of sodium excretion. *Renin* is an enzyme produced by the kidneys in the juxtaglomerular apparatus of each nephron. Upon release into the circulation, renin acts upon a substrate globulin from the liver to produce *angiotensin I,* which consists of 10 amino acids. A converting enzyme in the lungs and other tissues cleaves two amino acids from angiotensin I to form *angiotensin II,* which is an extremely potent vasoconstrictor. Angiotensin II also stimulates the release of aldosterone from the adrenal cortex. Removal of an amino acid from angiotensin II produces another molecule with biological activity (angiotensin III) whose physiological role is still under study.

Retrograde Pyelogram.   An x-ray study of the ureter, renal pelvis, and its calyces. Before the films are taken, the ureter is catheterized from below with the help of an instrument (cystoscope) placed into the bladder. Iodine-containing contrast material is then injected into the ureter counter to the direction of urine flow (retrograde) until it fills the ureter and renal pelvis, allowing them to be visualized on roentgenograms. The study may be done on one or both sides. This examination is more difficult and more stressful than an intravenous pyelogram, but it provides better visualization of the ureters and is especially useful in patients with poor renal function.

Serum Sickness.   A disorder that occurs (usually after an interval of some days) following the injection of foreign protein. This condition is easily produced in the laboratory by injecting bovine serum albumin into rabbits and has therefore become a model for the study of immune-complex disease. Such laboratory studies have shown that active illness is related to the formation of immune complexes (consisting of the foreign protein and host antibodies against it) of a critical size and in large numbers. The deposition of these complexes in various tissues, such as skin, joints, and renal glomeruli, appears to cause the clinical manifestations of the disease.

Silver Stain.   A histochemical staining sequence that utilizes methenamine silver in addition to other reagents to stain basement membrane in glomerular capillaries and similar material in the mesangium. It is used in renal pathology to delineate glomerular deposits.

Specific Gravity.   The density of a solution in relation to the density of pure water. The specific gravity of urine is often used in clinical medicine as a measure of concentration or dilution (i.e., osmolality). Though this simple determination can be performed with very inexpensive equipment, it may be somewhat misleading if heavy molecules such as protein or contrast agents are present in the urine. Primarily for this reason the

urine osmolality is a more reliable indicator of urinary concentration/
dilution.

Starling Forces. The hydrostatic and oncotic pressures that govern the movement of fluid across capillary walls. Discussed on pages 4–6.

Third Factor. As explained on page 65, this term was formerly used in the literature to describe a determinant of renal sodium excretion other than the two factors known at the time. It appears now that third factor may actually be several mechanisms.

Threshold. As used in renal physiology, this term usually refers to the highest plasma concentration of a filterable substance that allows its complete resorption by the tubules. At plasma concentrations above threshold, resorptive capacity is no longer adequate to recover all of the substance from the tubular fluid, and some of it appears in the urine. This concept is used in connection with substances that are filtered but do not usually appear in the urine, such as glucose.

Titratable Acidity (TA). The amount of hydrogen ion the renal tubules have added to urinary buffers other than bicarbonate and ammonia. TA is measured by determining the milliequivalents of sodium hydroxide needed to titrate acid urine back to a pH of 7.4. Discussed on pages 96–97.

Total Body Water. The total amount of water in the body; the sum of intracellular and all extracellular water.

Transcellular Water (transcellular fluid). Body water contained in a number of separate specialized pools sequestered by active transport activity. See pages 2–3.

Transport Maximum (Tm). The maximum rate of active transport of a substance, given an excess of substrate. This concept may apply to both active resorptive and active secretory processes. As the available amount of a transported substance increases, the quantity transported also increases, but only up to a certain limit. At that point the transport system is said to be *saturated*, and availability of additional substrate will not increase the rate of active transport any further.

Ultrafiltration. A process of selective filtration in which large molecules such as proteins are prevented from passing through the filtration barrier, even though they are in true solution. Normal glomerular filtration is an example of ultrafiltration.

Ultrasonography. A diagnostic technique for defining structures within the body by means of reflected ultrasonic waves.

Uremia. A toxic clinical state associated with severe renal failure. See also **Azotemia.**

Urinary Sediment. Particulate matter in the urine that precipitates upon simple centrifugation and that can be examined by light microscopy. The finding in urinary sediment of red blood cells, white blood cells, epithelial cells, casts, crystals, or bacteria can provide useful information about the presence of disease in the urinary tract and its possible type and location.

Vasopressin.   See **Antidiuretic hormone.**

Vesicoureteral Reflux.   Back-flow of urine from the bladder into one or both ureters; this abnormality of function is most likely to occur when pressure in the bladder increases during micturition (urination).

Index

An asterisk (*) indicates that the term is in the Glossary.